Seasonal Ayurveda - Aligning Lifestyle with Nature Cycles

Author
Dr. Vivek B Singh
BAMS, MD, PhD (Sch)
Assistant Professor,
RKCAMS, Bhopal.

Editor
Dr. Supriya Kurane
BAMS, MS, PhD (Sch)
Institute of Teaching and Research of Ayurveda, Jamnagar.

Preface

Welcome to a journey through the ancient wisdom of Ayurveda, tailored to harmonize with the natural cycles of the seasons. This book, "Seasonal Ayurveda – Aligning Lifestyle with Nature's Cycles," aims to guide you through understanding and implementing Ayurvedic principles to enhance your health and well-being by syncing your lifestyle with the rhythmic patterns of nature.

Ayurveda, a traditional system of medicine from India, teaches that health is a balanced interaction between the environment, body, mind, and spirit. Central to this understanding is the concept of the doshas – Vata, Pitta, and Kapha – which are energies found throughout the human body and mind. These energies fluctuate according to the seasons, and thus, adjusting our lifestyle accordingly can help maintain balance and prevent disease.

This book unfolds the secrets of adapting your diet, exercise, and overall wellness practices as per seasonal changes to support the natural balance of your body. Whether it is the rejuvenating air of spring, the fiery heat of summer, the grounding energy of autumn, or the nourishing calm of winter, each season holds unique challenges and gifts for our health.

The aim here is not just to provide you with a series of steps but to immerse you in a way of life that brings you closer to nature's rhythms. Each chapter will include practical advice on managing dietary needs, choosing appropriate physical activities, and implementing daily and seasonal routines that resonate with Ayurvedic teachings. Additionally, you will find detailed descriptions of seasonal detox routines, recommended asanas, and dietary tips to align your body and mind with the ongoing seasonal energies.

In writing this book, I hope to bridge the ancient knowledge of Ayurveda with your day-to-day activities, making it accessible, understandable, and beneficial. Whether you are new to Ayurveda or looking to deepen your existing practice, this guide is designed to provide valuable insights that can be tailored to anyone's lifestyle.

Thank you for choosing to embark on this path with me. Let's embrace the wisdom of Ayurveda together and learn to live a life in harmonious alignment with nature.

By the end of this preface, readers should feel welcomed and prepared to explore how Ayurveda can help them attune to the energy of each season for optimum health and vitality.

-Dr Vivek Singh
BAMS, MD, PhD (Sch)

Foreword

In a world that increasingly leans towards quick fixes and instant gratification, the ancient wisdom of Ayurveda offers a refreshing, holistic approach to health and wellness that is as relevant today as it was thousands of years ago. "Seasonal Ayurveda – Aligning Lifestyle with Nature's Cycles" is a timely resource that bridges the profound insights of Ayurvedic medicine with the practical demands of modern lifestyles, guiding readers on how to harmonize their health practices with the rhythms of nature.

This book arrives at a crucial juncture, as more individuals seek sustainable, health-conscious practices that honor both the body's innate wisdom and the environment. Dr. Vivek Singh, a seasoned Ayurvedic practitioner and scholar, brings his extensive knowledge and experience to the table, offering readers a comprehensive guide that is both enlightening and accessible.

Drawing from his rich background in clinical practice and academic teaching, Dr. Singh adeptly translates complex Ayurvedic concepts into practical applications, making them accessible to everyone, from beginners to advanced practitioners. Each page of this book is infused with his passion for Ayurveda and his commitment to spreading this knowledge for the betterment of all.

As you turn these pages, you will discover how each season impacts your health and how adjusting your diet, exercise, and daily routines can help you avoid common seasonal maladies and enhance your overall well-being. This book not only provides the 'what' and 'how' but also delves into the 'why' of each practice, empowering you with a deeper understanding and appreciation of Ayurveda.

I am confident that "Seasonal Ayurveda – Aligning Lifestyle with Nature's Cycles" will serve as an invaluable resource for those looking to enrich their lives through Ayurvedic practices. It stands as a testament to Dr. Singh's dedication to fostering a healthier world through ancient wisdom, adapted for contemporary needs.

May this book inspire you to embrace the cyclical nature of life and find balance and health throughout the changing seasons.

Dr Supriya Kurane
BAMS, MS, PhD (Sch)
Institute of Teaching and Research in Ayurveda,
Jamnagar.
8th November 2024

Index

Introduction to Ayurveda

Ayurveda, which translates to "the science of life" in Sanskrit, is one of the world's oldest holistic healing systems. Developed more than 3,000 years ago in India, it is based on the belief that health and wellness depend on a delicate balance between the mind, body, and spirit. Its main goal is not just to fight diseases but to promote good health, and it does so by integrating and balancing these elements.

The Foundations of Ayurveda
At the heart of Ayurveda are the concepts of the Doshas: Vata, Pitta, and Kapha. These are the three fundamental energies or life forces that govern the physical and mental processes in every human being. Understanding and balancing these Doshas, according to Ayurveda, is key to maintaining health.

- Vata (Air and Space): Governs movement and communication within the body, including breathing, blood circulation, and thought processes. When balanced, Vata promotes creativity and flexibility, but excess can induce fear and anxiety.

- Pitta (Fire and Water): Oversees digestion and metabolism, body temperature, and intellectual processing. In balance, Pitta promotes understanding and intelligence, but an imbalance can cause anger and inflammation.

- Kapha (Water and Earth): Controls growth, strength, stability, weight, and the immune system. Balanced Kapha is expressed as love and forgiveness, whereas excess can lead to attachment and greed.

Ayurvedic Diagnostics and Treatments
Ayurvedic diagnostics are distinctive because they involve a comprehensive assessment of the individual using techniques such as pulse diagnosis, tongue diagnosis, and observation of physical form and facial features. Based on this assessment, an Ayurvedic practitioner can deduce the state of the Doshas and the specific imbalances to address.

Treatment in Ayurveda is personalized. It may include dietary changes, herbal supplements, yoga, meditation, detoxification programs (like Panchakarma), and various other lifestyle adjustments. The mark of Ayurvedic treatment is its focus on identification and rectification of the root cause of a problem, rather than just alleviating symptoms.

Philosophical and Ethical Context
Beyond the physical aspects, Ayurveda places a strong emphasis on ethical, philosophical, and spiritual dimensions of health. It teaches that humans should live in harmony not only within themselves but also with their environment. Practices such as Dinacharya (daily routines) and Ritucharya (seasonal routines) are recommended to help individuals align their internal system with the natural world.

Ayurveda Today

Although ancient, Ayurveda remains relevant in the modern world. Its integration with other traditional and modern health systems has garnered global interest, promoting a more holistic approach to healthcare. Many of its herbal treatments and lifestyle recommendations have been supported by scientific research, further validating its effectiveness.

By understanding and applying Ayurvedic principles, individuals can anticipate improved health outcomes characterized by a greater equilibrium between the body, mind, and surrounding environment. This book aims to delve into these principles, focusing specifically on how you can adapt your lifestyle according to each season to harness optimal health.

Importance of Aligning with Seasonal Cycles

In Ayurveda, the concept of aligning our lifestyle with the natural cycles of the seasons is deeply ingrained. Recognizing and adapting to these seasonal changes is crucial because the external environment significantly influences our internal balance of the doshas—Vata, Pitta, and Kapha. This section explains why it's essential to harmonize with these cycles and how doing so can enhance overall health and wellbeing.

1. Prevention of Disease:

Ayurveda teaches that most diseases result from an imbalance of the doshas; each season naturally aggravates or pacifies certain doshas. For instance, Vata can become aggravated during the dry and cool conditions of autumn, while Pitta may increase in the hot summer months, and Kapha accumulates during the cold, damp winter. By adjusting our diet, lifestyle, and routines in accordance with the season, we can prevent the excessive accumulation of these doshas, thereby preventing disease before it starts.

2. Optimal Physical Health:
Each season brings specific challenges; for example, winters can be harsh on the immune system, and summers can lead to dehydration. Ayurveda offers seasonal regimens (Ritucharya) which include dietary adjustments, tailored exercise routines, and detoxification processes (such as Panchakarma). These practices help sustain our body's built-in defences and enhance vitality, keeping the body strong and resilient against seasonal threats.

3. Enhanced Mental and Emotional Wellbeing:
Seasons don't just influence our physical health; they impact our mental and emotional states as well. The practice of aligning our lifestyles with the seasonal cycles helps mitigate mood swings and emotional disturbances that can occur due to the weather and its impact on our bodies. For instance, the practice of calming, grounding activities in autumn can help counterbalance the airiness of Vata, which if aggravated, may cause anxiety and restlessness.

4. Improved Digestion and Metabolism:
Each season impacts Agni (digestive fire) differently.
Summer heat can increase Pitta, thus boosting our
digestive capacity, whereas the cold of winter might
dampen it. By eating season-specific foods and
engaging in suitable physical activities, we can
maintain an optimal metabolic rate and efficient
digestion, which are key to good health.

5. Sustainability:
Seasonal living is inherently sustainable. It encourages
the consumption of locally available, seasonal
produce, reducing the ecological footprint associated
with transporting non-seasonal food. Moreover, plants
harvested in their appropriate seasons are likely to be
at peak nutritional value, which further supports good
health.

6. Harmonious Existence:
Finally, living in tune with the seasonal cycles fosters
a harmonious existence with nature. It increases our
awareness of our environment and helps us respect the
natural order, promoting not just individual well-being
but also the well-being of our planet.

By embracing the wisdom of Seasonal Ayurveda, we
learn to flow with the natural rhythms rather than
resist them, leading to a more balanced, healthy, and
fulfilling life. This book guides you through adjusting
your lifestyle with practical advice tailored for each
season, helping you achieve harmony and balance
throughout the year.

Chapter 1: Understanding the Doshas and Seasons

A. Overview of the three doshas—Vata, Pitta, and Kapha

Vata Dosha

Introduction to Vata

Vata is derived from the elements of Air and Space (Ether) and translates to "that which moves things." It is considered the most powerful of the three doshas because it governs the principle of movement and is the force behind the other two doshas, which are incapable of movement without it.

Characteristics of Vata

Physically, individuals with a predominant Vata constitution are often thin, tall or very short, with dry skin and hair, and cold hands and feet. They are quick thinkers but also tend to forget easily. Emotionally, when balanced, they are energetic, creative, and flexible. An imbalanced Vata can lead to anxiety, insomnia, dry skin, and digestive issues.

Classical Shloka on Vata (Ashtanga Hridayam – Sutrasthanam, chapter 1, verse 11)

"Rooksha Laghu Sheeta, Khara Sukshma Chalo Anila"

Translation:
"Vata is dry, light, cold, rough, subtle, and mobile."

This shloka highlights the inherent qualities of Vata, emphasizing its dry, light, and mobile nature, which impacts the physiological and psychological tendencies of Vata individuals.

Pitta Dosha

Introduction to Pitta
Pitta is composed of Fire and Water elements and translates to "that which digests things". Pitta governs all heat, metabolism, and transformation in the body, including digestion and absorption of nutrients as well as cellular metabolism.

Characteristics of Pitta
Pitta types are usually of medium build, muscular, and well-proportioned. They have warm bodies, can be intense and goal-oriented, and may have a sharp wit. Their skin can be fair or reddish, often with freckles; they tend to have premature greying or thinning of hair. Balanced Pitta individuals are bright and intelligent. When out of balance, they can be overly critical, hot-tempered, and suffer from inflammatory conditions.

Classical Shloka on Pitta (Ashtanga Hridayam – Sutrasthanam, chapter 1, verse 10)

"Sasneha tikshnoshna, laghu visram, sara dravam"

Translation:
"Pitta is slightly oily, sharp, hot, light, foul-smelling, spreading and liquid."

This verse underlines the sharp, hot nature of Pitta, explaining its capacity to spread, and its penetrating qualities, which contribute to its role in transformational processes in the body.

Kapha Dosha

Introduction to Kapha
Derived from Water and Earth elements, Kapha is what binds the cells together, forming muscle, fat, bone, and sinew. It provides the structures and lubrication the body needs. The term Kapha translates to "that which sticks".

Characteristics of Kapha
Kapha types tend to have a sturdier, heavier build, are strong and can endure physical exertion. They have smooth, oily skin, thick wavy hair, and are particularly good-natured, calm, and easygoing when in balance. An excess of Kapha can lead to lethargy, weight gain, congestion, and resistance to change.

Classical Shloka on Kapha (Ashtanga Hridayam – Sutrasthanam, chapter 1, verse 12)

"Snigdho guru manda, Shlakshno Mrutsna Sthira Kapha"

"Kapha is unctuous, heavy, slow, smooth, soft, and stable."

This shloka articulates the heavy, slow yet stable nature of Kapha that contributes to growth, cohesion, and stability within the biological system.

Integration in Ayurvedic Diagnosis and Treatment
Understanding Vata, Pitta, and Kapha involves not just an analysis of their properties and effects when in balance or imbalance but also the appropriate integration of this knowledge in lifestyle management and therapeutic interventions. An experienced Ayurvedic practitioner assesses the predominant dosha(s) and the state of doshic imbalance before recommending a personalized treatment regime. This holistic approach can include dietary changes, herbal supplements, body treatments, yoga asanas, meditation, and lifestyle adjustments specific to each individual's prakriti (natural constitution) and vikriti (imbalanced state).

B. <u>Seasons and Their Corresponding Doshas</u>

In Ayurveda, the concept of Ritucharya, or seasonal regimen, underscores the profound link between the cycles of nature and human health. Just as the seasons impact the environment directly, they also influence the balance of doshas — the fundamental bio-energies

18

of Vata, Pitta, and Kapha — within the human body. Each season tends to aggravate or pacify certain doshas, thus impacting our health in different ways. Understanding which doshas are prominent in each season helps to tailor diet, exercise, and overall lifestyle to maintain harmony and health throughout the year.

Spring (Vasanta)
- Primary Dosha: Kapha
- Characteristics: As snow melts and the weather warms, Kapha, which has accumulated during the cold and wet winter months, begins to liquefy and move through the body. This can lead to a feeling of heaviness, and if not managed, may result in colds, sinus congestion, or allergies.
- Ayurvedic Focus: To counterbalance the increase in Kapha, it's advised to embrace a warming and drying diet that includes foods like honey, ginger, and pulses. Activities should be more vigorous to shake off winter sluggishness. Spring is also an ideal time for cleansing and detoxification routines like Panchakarma.

Summer (Grishma)
- Primary Dosha: Pitta
- Characteristics: The heat of summer increases Pitta, leading to enhanced metabolic and digestive activity. Pitta's fire can lead to irritability, excessive body heat, and inflammatory conditions if it becomes excessive.
- Ayurvedic Focus: Cooling measures are essential. Diets should include sweet, bitter, and astringent tastes — think fresh fruits, vegetables, and dairy products. It's also beneficial to engage in cooling

exercises, such as swimming and moonlit walks. Drinking plenty of fluids and the use of cooling oils like coconut oil for the skin are recommended.

Monsoon/Rainy Season (Varsha)
- Primary Dosha: Vata
- Characteristics: The end of summer leads into the monsoon, and this sudden change in weather can disrupt Vata, which is characterized by qualities of movement and change. Vata imbalances manifest as dry skin, anxiety, irregular digestion, and joint pain.
- Ayurvedic Focus: The diet should be stabilizing and nourishing, including foods that are sweet, salty, and sour. Warm soups, cooked grains like rice and wheat, and spiced teas are beneficial. It's also a good time for gentle massages with sesame oil to keep Vata grounded.

Autumn (Sharad)
- Primary Dosha: Pitta
- Characteristics: In many regions, autumn is a pitta-aggravating season due to the continuing warmth and decreasing humidity, which can trigger skin issues, acid reflux, and hot tempers.
- Ayurvedic Focus: Similar to summer, maintaining a cooling regimen is advised with an emphasis on bitter, astringent, and sweet tastes. Invigorating morning practices like yoga can be beneficial to balance the body's energy.

Early Winter (Hemanta)
- Primary Dosha: Vata

- Characteristics: Cold and dry qualities of early winter exacerbate Vata. This can lead to increased mental stress, physical dryness (skin, hair), and discomfort in the joints.
- Ayurvedic Focus: Diet should focus on nourishing and hydrating foods — nuts, seeds, root vegetables, and fatty fruits like avocados. Warm, spiced (not spicy) foods are ideal. Physical activity should be moderate and warming, and hydration is crucial.

Late Winter to Early Spring (Shishira)
- Primary Dosha: Kapha
- Characteristics: As winter deepens, colder temperatures continue to aggravate Kapha leading to colds, coughs, and a feeling of lethargy.
- Ayurvedic Focus: Foods that are warming and light help counter dampness, and physical activity should be invigorated to stoke the internal heat and keep the lymph moving. Spices such as cinnamon, clove, and black pepper are especially good during this time.

By tailoring daily habits and diets to these seasonal needs, Ayurveda empowers individuals to maintain balance and health all year round. Each season's regime helps prepare the body for the next, ensuring smooth transitions and reducing the chances of seasonal illnesses.

C. <u>How Seasons Affect Our Health</u>

Understanding how the changing seasons affect our health is a fundamental aspect of Ayurveda, a holistic approach that promotes harmony between body, mind, and environment. Each season brings unique external conditions (temperature, humidity, wind, etc.), influencing the balance of the three primary doshas (Vata, Pitta, and Kapha) within the body. The seasonal variations can significantly impact physical health, emotional well-being, and overall vitality.

How Seasonal Changes Impact Health:

1. Temperature Shifts:

Each dosha responds differently to temperature changes. Vata is cold and dry, so the cold seasons can aggravate it, leading to dry skin, stiffness in joints, and digestive issues. Pitta is hot, so during warmer seasons, there might be an increase in body heat leading to skin irritations, acidity, and temper flare-ups. Kapha is cool and moist, predominant during late winter and spring; excess can lead to colds, sinus congestion, and lethargy.

2. Humidity and Dryness:

Humidity increases Kapha, which can cause heaviness, sluggishness, and excess mucus production. Dry conditions elevate Vata, often leading to dry skin, hair, and nails, as well as vulnerability to nervous system disorders and anxiety. An optimal balance is needed to handle these impacts, and Ayurveda recommends season-specific routines to maintain such balance.

3. Daylight Variations:

Longer days in summer can increase activity levels, boosting metabolism and overall energy. Conversely, shorter days in winter can increase melatonin production, encouraging more sleep and less activity, which can increase Kapha and decrease Vata and Pitta. Seasonal Affective Disorder (SAD) is a clear example of how reduced sunlight exposure can affect mood and energy levels.

4. Dietary Influence:
Seasonal fruits and vegetables provide the nutrients most needed for that time of the year. For instance, summer fruits like watermelon and cucumber help hydrate the body and cool down the internal heat, beneficial during Pitta-aggravating seasons. In contrast, root vegetables available during the winter provide deeper nourishment and grounding which is perfect for balancing the elevated Vata.

5. Allergens:
Seasonal changes, especially from winter to spring, can spike pollen levels, affecting those susceptible to allergies. The increase of Kapha in spring can exacerbate these issues, resulting in symptoms such as sneezing, congestion, and headaches.

6. Mental and Emotional Health:
The connection between the season and mental health is profound. Winter can induce feelings of depression and lethargy (enhanced Kapha), while spring might renew energy and creativity. Understanding one's dosha can help predict and mitigate these mental shifts with appropriate lifestyle adjustments.

Ayurvedic Recommendations for Seasonal Health:
To mitigate the effects of seasonal changes and maintain dosha balance, Ayurveda suggests specific lifestyle adjustments:
- Diet: Eat season-appropriate foods that balance the dominant dosha. For example, adding spicy or warm foods in winter to balance Kapha and Vata, and cooling foods in summer for Pitta.
- Exercise: Varying exercise intensity according to the season; more calming and less strenuous exercises like yoga and swimming in summer, and more vigorous activities in winter to stimulate heat and energy.
- Routine: Adjusting waking and sleeping times to sync with sunrise and sunset, benefiting from natural light as much as possible.
- Detoxification: Engaging in Panchakarma (an Ayurvedic detoxifying process) during seasonal transitions to cleanse accumulated doshas and rejuvenate the body.
- Mindfulness and Meditation: Practicing mindfulness and meditation can help maintain emotional and mental balance throughout seasonal shifts.

Acknowledging and adapting to these seasonal influences can significantly enhance well-being by promoting balance both internally and externally, illustrating Ayurveda's profound connection between nature's rhythms and human health.

Chapter 2: Spring (Vasant) - Renewal and Rejuvenation

A. Overview of Spring Characteristics and Dietary Needs

Spring is a vibrant time of renewal and regrowth, both in the natural world and within our bodies. According to Ayurveda, spring is predominantly associated with the Kapha dosha, which is characterized by qualities of heaviness, coldness, and moisture. This season sees the melting of winter's accumulation of snow and ice, paralleling the body's natural inclination to liquefy and lighten the accumulated cold and heavy Kapha of winter.

Characteristics of Spring:
- Temperature: Generally mild but can fluctuate between cool mornings and evenings to warm mid-days.
- Humidity: Increased moisture in the air with frequent rain or damp conditions, aiding plant growth.
- Growth: Energetic blooming and sprouting of plants and flowers, symbolizing renewal.
- Living Beings: Increased activity in animals coming out of hibernation and higher human energy levels post-winter.

Health Impact:
During spring, the accumulated Kapha begins to liquefy, leading to higher risks of colds, flu, allergies,

and sinus congestion. People may also experience a feeling of heaviness, sluggish digestion, and water retention. However, properly managing Kapha during this time can lead to revitalization and great vitality.

Dietary Needs for Spring:
The key to balancing Kapha in spring is to focus on foods that are light, warm, and dry, which counteract its cold, heavy, and moist qualities. Here are specific dietary guidelines for optimizing health during spring:

1. Favor Light and Warm Foods:
- Opt for warm, cooked foods instead of cold or raw items. Light broths, soups, and steamed vegetables can be very suitable.
- Incorporate warming spices like ginger, black pepper, cumin, and turmeric in your meals to help boost digestion and metabolism.

2. Emphasize Bitter, Pungent, and Astringent Tastes:
- Bitter greens like kale, dandelion, and arugula help cleanse the body of excess Kapha.
- Pungent flavours such as chillies, radishes, onions, and garlic aid in heating and drying the body, which is beneficial to counteract the moist and heavy qualities of spring.
- Astringent foods like legumes, green apples, and pomegranate help absorb water, tighten tissues and dry out excess moisture.

3. Reduce Heavy and Oily Foods:

- Decrease the intake of dairy products, which can exacerbate mucus production.
- Avoid fried foods and meats that are high in fat as they are harder to digest and can contribute to sluggishness.

4. Incorporate Grains and Beans:
- Grains like barley, quinoa, and millet are light and easy to digest, making them excellent choices for spring.
- Beans are also beneficial as they are dry and astringent, which helps balance Kapha's oily nature.

5. Hydration:
- While hydration is essential, avoid very cold or chilled beverages as they can dampen the digestive fire (Agni).
- Opt for room temperature or warm water, possibly with a slice of lemon or a pinch of cayenne for its cleansing effects.

6. Herbal Teas:
- Herbal teas like ginger tea, green tea, or Tulsi tea can be useful for stimulating metabolism and reducing water retention.

By aligning your diet with the needs of the season, you can effectively manage Kapha, boost your immunity, enhance your digestion, and enjoy the revitalizing energy of spring. This not only prepares the body for the upcoming warmer months but also optimizes health and well-being during this transitional season.

B. <u>Detoxifying the Body – Spring Cleanse</u>

Spring is an ideal time for cleansing and revitalization. In Ayurveda, this season is associated with the Kapha dosha, which can accumulate throughout the winter and manifest as excess weight, lethargy, or congestion as the weather starts to warm. A spring cleanse aims to rejuvenate the body by eliminating these accumulated toxins (ama) and balancing Kapha, thereby enhancing vitality and overall health.

Purpose of Spring Cleanse
The primary goals of a spring cleanse in Ayurvedic practice are to:
- Clear the channels of the body of excess Kapha and ama.
- Revitalize the digestive system to boost metabolism.
- Enhance the body's natural immunity.
- Promote overall balance and well-being.

Elements of a Spring Cleanse
1. Simplified Diet
The cornerstone of a spring cleanse is a simplified, light diet that is easy to digest. This typically includes:
   - Kitchari: A traditional Ayurvedic dish made from mung beans and basmati rice with spices like turmeric, cumin, coriander, and fennel to stimulate the digestive fire (Agni) without overwhelming it.

- Steamed Vegetables: Light and fibrous vegetables like carrots, celery, beets, and leafy greens that promote bowel movement and detoxification.
- Fruits: Especially those that are astringent or bitter such as apples, pears, and berries.
- Consumption should focus on foods with bitter, astringent, and pungent tastes to help reduce Kapha's heavy and sticky qualities.

2. Drink Plenty of Fluids
- Warm Water: Regular sipping of warm water throughout the day helps to flush out toxins and keeps the hydration levels up without dampening the digestive fire.
- Herbal Teas: Teas made from ginger, dandelion, nettle, or burdock root help support liver function and assist in the removal of toxins.

3. Lifestyle Adjustments
- Daily Exercise: Light to moderate activities such as walking, yoga, and stretching help keep the lymph moving and assist in clearing out toxins. Focus on yoga poses that stimulate the abdominal area to enhance digestion.
- Adequate Sleep: Ensure to get enough rest as the body heals and rejuvenates itself during sleep.

4. Ayurvedic Therapies
- Abhyanga (Ayurvedic Oil Massage): A self-massage with warm oil, such as sesame for Kapha, helps improve circulation and calms the nervous system.

- Steam Therapy (Swedana): After oil massage, taking a warm bath or steam bath can help to open the pores and channels of the body, allowing toxins to flow out more easily.

- Nasya: Administration of herbal oils into the nostrils to cleanse accumulated Kapha in the sinuses and head.

5. Herbal Supplements

- Triphala: A well-known Ayurvedic blend those aids in cleansing the digestive tract and ensuring regular bowel movements.

- Tulsi: Known for its detoxifying and immune-boosting properties.

- Guggulu: Useful for its purifying and rejuvenating properties.

Precautions

Before beginning any cleanse, especially a rigorous one, it's advisable to consult with an Ayurvedic practitioner, particularly for individuals with specific health conditions or those who are pregnant or nursing.

A spring cleanse is fundamentally about giving the body a chance to reset and refresh. By reducing the intake of heavy foods, introducing light and nourishing alternatives, and adopting cleansing practices, your body can shed the sluggishness of winter. This allows for a rejuvenated start to the season with heightened energy levels and improved well-being.

C. <u>Spring-Specific Asanas and Exercise Routines</u>

Spring is an ideal time for invigorating the body through yoga and exercise, especially to counteract the heavy and stagnant qualities of Kapha that can accumulate during the winter months. In Ayurveda, spring exercises are designed to be lightening, warming, and drying to balance the Kapha dosha. Here are several yoga asanas and exercise routines specifically recommended for the spring season to stimulate circulation, boost metabolism, and enhance overall vitality.

Yoga Asanas for Spring

1. Sun Salutations (Surya Namaskar):
   This dynamic sequence warms up the body, enhances cardiovascular fitness, and improves the efficiency of the respiratory system. Its rhythmic, flowing movements help to break up stagnation and energize the entire body.

2. Twisting Poses (Ardha Matsyendrasana - Half Lord of the Fishes Pose):
   Twists are excellent for stimulating digestion and helping with the detoxification processes. They squeeze out toxins from the abdominal organs and promote fresh blood flow to those areas upon release.

3. Backbends (Bhujangasana - Cobra Pose, Ustrasana - Camel Pose):

Backbends open up the chest and lungs, increase spinal flexibility, and can help clear out phlegm from the respiratory tract, making them particularly useful for reducing Kapha.

4. Standing Poses (Ardha Chandrasana - Half Moon Pose, Virabhadrasana - Warrior Pose):
These poses strengthen and tone the body, improve balance and stamina, and increase bodily heat, which helps to dry out excess Kapha.

5. Breath-Linked Movement and Pranayama (Kapalbhati - Skull Shining Breath):
Practices such as Kapalbhati are not only invigorating but also cleansing for the respiratory system. This type of breath work helps to expel old, stagnant air from the lungs, enhance lung capacity, and generate internal heat.

Exercise Routines for Spring
1. Brisk Walking or Jogging:
Cardiovascular activities like fast-paced walking or jogging are ideal for spring. They invigorate the circulatory system and reduce lethargy and depression by boosting endorphin production.

2. Circuit Training:
Short bursts of different exercises (e.g., jumping jacks, squats, push-ups) help keep the workout dynamic and engaging, promoting strength and endurance without overtaxing the body.

3. Biking or Swimming:
   These are also excellent ways to get both an aerobic workout and muscular toning without the high impact on joints that can aggravate Vata.

Incorporating Movement into Daily Routine
1. Morning Routine:
   Starting the day with a light stretching routine or a few rounds of Sun Salutations can help kickstart the metabolism and maintain balanced energy levels throughout the day.

2. Break Up Sedentary Periods:
   Taking short breaks during long periods of inactivity (like working at a desk) to stretch or do a quick set of exercises can help maintain energy and prevent the accumulation of Kapha.

3. Outdoor Activities:
   Engaging in outdoor activities can also be beneficial due to the exposure to fresh air and sunlight, which are invigorating for the body and mind, further helping to alleviate springtime lethargy.

These yoga asanas and exercise routines, individuals can effectively manage the seasonal transition into spring, reducing Kapha accumulation, enhancing detoxification, and improving overall vitality and health. Always ensure to listen to your body and adjust the intensity of your activities to match your current health condition and fitness level.

D. Recipes for Spring – Balancing Kapha

During spring, the primary goal for maintaining a balanced diet in Ayurveda is to mitigate the typical accumulation of Kapha dosha. This involves incorporating foods that are light, warm, and dry, and favouring tastes that are bitter, pungent, and astringent. Below are a few recipes that embody these principles, helping to invigorate the body and alleviate the heavy and moist qualities of Kapha.

1. Detoxifying Kitchari
Ingredients:
- 1/2 cup basmati rice
- 1 cup mung dal (split yellow)
- 6 cups (approx.) water
- 1/2 to 1 inch ginger root, chopped or grated
- A pinch of mineral salt (adjust to taste)
- 2 tsp. turmeric powder
- 2 tsp. coriander powder
- 2 tsp. cumin powder
- 1/2 tsp. whole mustard seeds
- 1/2 tsp. fennel seeds
- 1 handful fresh cilantro leaves, chopped
- 1 cup assorted vegetables (such as carrot, celery, or zucchini), chopped
- 2 tbsp. ghee (clarified butter)

Instructions:

1. Wash the rice and mung dal and soak overnight, if possible, then drain.

2. In a medium saucepan or a large skillet, heat the ghee over medium heat. Add mustard seeds, cumin seeds, and fennel seeds, sauté until they start to pop.

3. Add the turmeric, coriander, cumin powders, and ginger into the ghee and stir them together.

4. Add rice, mung dal, and vegetables to the mixture and stir again.

5. Pour in 6 cups of water and bring it to a boil. Once boiling, reduce heat to a simmer and cover, cooking until both the rice and dal are mushy (approximately 30-45 minutes).

6. Garnish with fresh cilantro and season with salt before serving.

This meal is light yet nourishing and perfect for balancing Kapha, with its combination of spices stimulating digestion.

2. Ginger Lemon Tea

Ingredients:
- 1-inch piece of fresh ginger, peeled and sliced thin
- 4 cups water
- Juice from 1/2 lemon
- Honey to taste (optional, use sparingly)

Instructions:
1. Boil the ginger slices in water for at least 10 minutes.

2. Remove from heat and add the lemon juice. Stir well.

3. Strain the tea into a cup and add honey if desired for a touch of sweetness.

This tea is excellent for stimulating agni (digestive fire) without increasing Pitta too much. It is warming and Kapha-pacifying.

3. Bitter Greens Salad with Lemon Vinaigrette

Ingredients for Salad:
- A mix of bitter greens such as kale, arugula, and dandelion greens
- 1/2 cup sliced radishes
- 1/4 cup pumpkin seeds

Ingredients for Lemon Vinaigrette:
- 1/4 cup olive oil
- Juice of 1 lemon
- 1 garlic clove, minced
- Salt and pepper to taste

Instructions:
1. Wash the greens and toss them with the sliced radishes in a large salad bowl.
2. In a small bowl, whisk together the olive oil, lemon juice, minced garlic, salt, and pepper.
3. Pour the vinaigrette over the salad and toss until evenly coated.
4. Sprinkle with pumpkin seeds before serving.

This salad is refreshing, with the bitterness of the greens helping to cleanse accumulated Kapha and the radishes providing a pleasant pungent kick.

These spring recipes are designed to combat the sluggishness often felt during Kapha season, boosting digestion and invigorating the body. Enjoy them as part of a balanced Ayurvedic spring routine to maintain health and vitality.

Chapter 3: Summer (Grishma) - Cooling and Soothing

A. Overview of Summer Characteristics and Dietary Needs

In Ayurveda, the summer season is predominantly governed by the Pitta dosha, which is composed of fire and water. This dosha influences the body's metabolic systems, including digestion, absorption of nutrients, and body temperature. The warmest season of the year, summer is characterized by increased heat, which can aggravate Pitta, leading to imbalances if not properly managed.

Characteristics of Summer:

- Temperature: Typically, the hottest period of the year, with long, sunny days.
- Humidity: Varies widely; some regions may experience dry spells, while others could have high humidity, especially in coastal or tropical areas.
- Sunlight: Increased daylight hours with intense sun exposure.
- Natural Environment: Flourishing flora and active fauna, a time of growth and maturation for many plants and animals.

Health Impact:

Excess Pitta during the summer can manifest in the body as skin irritations (like rashes and sunburn), inflammation, excessive body heat, and emotional imbalances such as irritability or anger. Digestive issues like hyperacidity, indigestion, or diarrhoea can also occur if Pitta is overly stimulated.

Dietary Needs for Summer:
The diet in summer should aim to balance the excess heat and provide hydration to prevent the aggravation of Pitta. Here's what typically works in aligning with the seasonal needs:

1. Favor Cooling Foods:
- Fruits: Watermelon, cucumbers, sweet berries, grapes, and pears are excellent to hydrate and cool down the body.
- Vegetables: Leafy greens, zucchini, pumpkins, broccoli, asparagus, and bell peppers are beneficial due to their high-water content and cooling properties.
- Dairy: Moderate use of dairy products like ghee, milk, unsweetened yogurt, and fresh cheese can also cool the body. These should be consumed in their natural or slightly cooled forms but not icy cold as it dampens the digestive fire.

2. Include Sweet, Bitter, and Astringent Tastes:
- These tastes are cooling and can balance Pitta. Herbs and spices like fennel, coriander, cardamom, and mint are excellent for their cooling effects. Avoid or minimize hot, spicy, and acidic condiments which can exacerbate Pitta.

3. Maintain Hydration:

- Drinks: Avoid icy beverages as they can inhibit digestion and instead opt for cool or room temperature drinks. Coconut water is particularly good for hydration and balancing electrolytes. Herbal teas like chamomile, peppermint, or hibiscus can be refreshing.
- Liquids Over Caffeine and Alcohol: These can dehydrate the body, so it's better to limit their consumption during hot months.

4. Cooking Methods:

- Opt for gentle cooking methods such as boiling, steaming, or poaching which do not contribute extra heat to the food. Raw foods are also applicable in moderation, especially during the peak heat when digestion is naturally stronger.

5. Time of Eating:

- Have your main meal at noon when the digestive fire (Agni) is strongest. Dinner should be lighter and eaten well before bedtime to ensure a night of cooler, more restful sleep.

Summer is a time when balancing the intrinsic heat with cooling elements becomes critical to maintain health. Adjusting dietary habits according to Ayurvedic principles helps in managing the Pitta dosha effectively, ensuring a season of vitality, and keeping heat-induced ailments at bay. These adjustments also align with enjoying the bounty of fruits and vegetables that nature provides specifically during these warmer months.

B. <u>Managing Heat with Ayurveda</u>

Managing heat effectively is crucial during the warmer months, especially when Pitta dosha, which encompasses the fire and water elements, becomes predominant. Ayurveda offers valuable insights and practices for cooling down internally, which can help in balancing Pitta during high temperatures. This can prevent the common summer complaints such as excessive body heat, inflammation, skin issues, and irritability. Here are several Ayurvedic strategies to manage heat and maintain a balanced state:

1. Dietary Adjustments

Ayurveda emphasizes the importance of diet in balancing doshas. To counteract the heat of Pitta: Emphasize Cooling Foods: Incorporate foods with cooling properties such as cucumbers, sweet fruits (like melons, grapes, pears, and mangoes), coconut, and ghee. Vegetables like zucchini, lettuce, and asparagus also have cooling effects.

Favor Sweet, Bitter, and Astringent Tastes: These tastes are known to calm Pitta. Good choices include salads with bitter greens, dals (lentils) seasoned with fresh herbs, and dishes flavoured with fennel, coriander, cardamom, and mint.

Reduce Spicy Foods: Minimize hot spices, sour fruits, and salty foods, which exacerbate Pitta. Instead of chili, opt for milder spices such as turmeric, black pepper, saffron, and cinnamon.

Stay Hydrated: Drink ample fluids, including cool (not ice cold) water infused with slices of cucumber or lime. Herbal teas like peppermint, liquorice root, or hibiscus are excellent for cooling the body and are gentle on the stomach.

2. Lifestyle Practices

Wear Light Colours and Fabrics: Colors like white, blue, green, and grey have cooling effects. Cotton and other natural Fibers help the body breathe and stay cool.

Time Your Activities: Engage in outdoor physical activities during the cooler parts of the day, such as early mornings or late afternoons. Avoid vigorous activity during the peak heat to prevent overheating.

Cooling Baths: Taking cool (not cold) showers or baths can help lower body temperature. Adding rose water or essential oils such as sandalwood or jasmine to bath water can also enhance the cooling effect.

3. Yoga and Breathing Practices

Practice Cooling Yoga Practices: Poses like Forward Bends, Moon Salutations, and Camel pose can be beneficial. Incorporate plenty of seated and supine poses that promote relaxation and cooling.

Sheetali Pranayama (Cooling Breath): This breathing technique has a cooling effect on the body and is very beneficial during hot weather. To practice, curl the tongue into a tube, inhale through the mouth, hold the breath for a few seconds, then close the mouth and exhale through the nose.

Meditation and Relaxation: Stress can exacerbate Pitta. Practices that promote mental calmness and emotional coolness are beneficial. Meditative practices that focus on the cooling lunar energy are recommended.

4. Herbs and Supplements
Aloe Vera: Known for its cooling properties, drinking aloe vera juice can help soothe the digestive tract and cool down the body.

Amalaki: Also known as Indian gooseberry, Amalaki is a potent rejuvenative that benefits the liver and cools down the body's internal heat.

Neem: Useful for its cooling and detoxifying properties; it helps in cleansing the blood and supporting clear skin.

5. Avoid Excessive Sun Exposure:
Limit direct exposure to the sun especially during peak times (10 AM to 4 PM). Using natural sunscreen and wearing a hat and sunglasses can protect the skin and eyes from the harsh effects of the sun.

By integrating these Ayurvedic principles and practices into your daily routine, you can effectively manage the increase in heat during the summer months, thereby reducing the risk of Pitta-related health issues.

C. Summer-Specific Asanas and Cooling Practices

During the summer months, when the heat intensity increases and Pitta dosha can become aggravated, it's beneficial to engage in yoga practices that are cooling and soothing. These practices can help manage the body's internal temperature, maintain a calm mind, and foster emotional balance. Here are some summer-specific asanas and cooling practices that are particularly effective:

Cooling Yoga Asanas

1.   Moon Salutation (Chandra Namaskar)
Unlike the more heating Sun Salutations, Moon Salutations are cooling and soothing. They include a series of poses that are performed in a flowing sequence at a slow and gentle pace. This practice honours the lunar qualities associated with cooling, receptiveness, and calmness.

2.   Forward Bends (Paschimottanasana, Uttanasana)
Forward bends are cooling and help calm the mind and reduce stress. They compress the abdomen slightly, which also aids in soothing the digestive system—a common seat of Pitta disturbance.

3.   Camel Pose (Ustrasana)

Gentle backbends like Camel Pose can open up the chest and cool the body. However, ensure not to overdo backbends as they can also stimulate heat if performed intensely or held for too long.

4.   Fish Pose (Matsyasana)
This pose stretches the chest and throat, areas often affected by excess heat. It helps open up respiratory channels, encouraging deep, cooling breaths.

5.   Supine Bound Angle Pose (Supta Baddha Konasana)
A restorative pose that allows for relaxation and cooling. The position opens up the hips and groin and can help release heat from the body.

6.   Legs Up the Wall (Viparita Karani)
This gentle inversion is excellent for cooling down and relaxing the entire system. It promotes circulation, eases swollen feet (common in heat), and calms the nervous system.

Cooling Pranayama (Breathing Exercises)
1. Sheetali Pranayama (Cooling Breath)
This breathing technique involves inhaling through a rolled tongue (or pursed lips if the tongue can't be rolled), holding the breath for a moment, and then slowly exhaling through the nose. The air taken in over the tongue has a cooling effect on the body.

2. Sitkari Pranayama

Similar to Sheetali, Sitkari involves inhaling through clenched teeth, holding the breath, and then exhaling slowly through the nose. It helps cool the body and calm the mind.

Cooling Practices and Lifestyle Adjustments

1. Practice During Cooler Parts of the Day
   Avoid practicing during the peak heat times (generally from 10 AM to 4 PM). Early morning or late evening are ideal times for yoga and physical activities.

2. Use Aromatherapy
   Essential oils such as sandalwood, rose, jasmine, and lavender have cooling effects. Use these in diffusers during your practice or apply them topically in a diluted form for a calming effect.

3. Drink Plenty of Fluids
   Hydration is crucial. Consume ample water, coconut water, or herbal teas to keep hydrated. Avoid ice-cold beverages as they can disrupt digestion according to Ayurvedic principles.

4. Wear Appropriate Clothing
   Wear loose, breathable fabrics in light colours to help reflect heat and allow your body to breathe during your practice.

Incorporating these summer-specific asanas and cooling practices into your daily routine can help you manage the summer heat more effectively, keeping

Pitta in balance and ensuring physical, mental, and emotional well-being through the hotter months.

D. Recipes for Summer – Pacifying Pitta

During the hot summer months, balancing Pitta dosha is crucial to maintain internal coolness and hydration. Consuming foods that are sweet, bitter, and astringent helps counteract the heat and acidity often exacerbated by summer. Here are some recipes that incorporate these qualities to help keep Pitta in balance during the season.

1. Cucumber Mint Salad
Ingredients:
- 2 large cucumbers peeled and thinly sliced.
- 1/4 cup freshly chopped mint leaves.
- 2 tablespoons lime juice
- 1 tablespoon olive oil
- Pink Himalayan salt, to taste
- Fresh ground black pepper, to taste
- Optional: 1/4 cup thinly sliced red onion

Instructions:
1. In a mixing bowl, combine the cucumber slices and chopped mint.
2. Drizzle with olive oil and lime juice. Mix gently.
3. Season with salt and pepper to taste. Add sliced red onion if using.
4. Chill in the refrigerator for at least 30 minutes before serving to allow the flavours to meld.

This salad is hydrating and refreshing, making it perfect for cooling down and pacifying Pitta.

2. Coconut Rice with Cardamom
Ingredients:
- 1 cup basmati rice, rinsed.
- 1 can (13.5 ounces) coconut milk
- 1/2 cup water
- 1 teaspoon cardamom powder
- 1/4 teaspoon salt
- 1 tablespoon coconut oil
- Optional: 1/2 cup toasted coconut flakes for garnish

Instructions:
1. In a saucepan, heat the coconut oil over medium heat.
2. Add the rinsed basmati rice and toast lightly for about 1-2 minutes.
3. Pour in the coconut milk and water, then add the cardamom and salt.
4. Bring to a boil, then reduce heat to low, cover, and simmer for 18-20 minutes, or until the liquid is absorbed and the rice is tender.
5. Remove from heat and let sit, covered, for 5 minutes.
6. Fluff with a fork and garnish with toasted coconut flakes if desired.
Coconut and cardamom both have cooling properties that are excellent for pacifying Pitta.

3. Green Mango Drink (Aam Panna)
Ingredients:
- 2 green mangoes

- 1/2 teaspoon roasted cumin powder
- 1/4 teaspoon cardamom powder
- Sugar or jaggery to taste
- A pinch of salt
- Mint leaves for garnish
- Ice cubes (optional)

Instructions:
1. Boil the mangoes in water until they become soft and the skin cracks. Let them cool.
2. Peel the mangoes and extract the pulp with a spoon.
3. Add the pulp to a blender along with sugar (or jaggery), cumin powder, cardamom, and salt. Blend until smooth.
4. Pour the mixture through a sieve into a large pitcher.
5. Add 2-3 cups of cold water to the pitcher and stir well.
6. Serve with ice cubes and garnish with mint leaves.

This drink is not only refreshing but also revitalizing due to the presence of mango, which is rich in vitamins and cooling spices.

4. Bitter Greens with Almonds and Lemon Dressing

Ingredients:
- 4 cups mixed bitter greens (e.g., kale, arugula, dandelion greens)
- 1/3 cup sliced almonds, toasted.
- For the dressing:
- 2 tablespoons lemon juice
- 1/4 cup extra virgin olive oil.

- 1 teaspoon Dijon mustard
- 1 garlic clove, minced.
- Salt and pepper to taste

Instructions:
1. Prepare the dressing by whisking together lemon juice, olive oil, Dijon mustard, minced garlic, salt, and pepper until well combined.
2. Place the greens in a large salad bowl.
3. Drizzle the dressing over the greens and toss until evenly coated.
4. Sprinkle toasted almonds on top before serving.

Bitter greens help cleanse the body and balance Pitta, while almonds add a nourishing, cooling effect beneficial for hot months.

These summer recipes focus on cooling, hydration, and the calming of Pitta fire, making them ideal for maintaining balance and wellness in the warmer season.

Chapter 4: Autumn (Sharad) - Grounding and Stabilization

A. Overview of Autumn Characteristics and Dietary Needs

Autumn, known as "Sharad", in Ayurveda, is a significant season characterized by a gradual shift from the hot, light, and intense qualities of summer to the cool, dry, and windy atmosphere of early winter. In many climates, early autumn still retains enough warmth to continue aggravating Pitta, which has accumulated during the summer. Hence, the transition into autumn can often lead to increased Pitta-related imbalances if not properly managed.

Characteristics of Autumn:
- Temperature: Although the intense heat of summer has passed, temperatures can still be warm, particularly in early autumn. This residual warmth can keep Pitta dosha high.
- Humidity: There's often less humidity in the air, which can start increasing Vata but may still hold enough moisture to aggravate Pitta.
- Wind: Increases as the season progresses, contributing to the dryness and coolness in the environment, initiating the gradual increase in Vata.

- Natural Phenomena: Leaves changing colours and falling are external signs of Pitta reducing and Vata increasing as the season advances.

Health Impact:
With Pitta having built up over the sunny months, the body can experience an overflow of Pitta's fire element, manifesting as:
- Skin Issues: Such as rashes, breakouts, or a flare-up of existing inflammatory skin conditions.
- Digestive Problems: Including acid reflux, ulcers, or diarrhoea, as Pitta governs the digestive fire (Agni).
- Emotional Distress: Irritability, frustration, and anger are typical signs of high Pitta.

Dietary Needs for Autumn:
To manage and pacify Pitta while accommodating the emerging Vata, one's diet in autumn requires a careful balance:

1. Favor Warm and Cooked Foods:
  - As the weather cools, the diet should shift from the cooling foods of summer to more warming dishes. Lightly cooked meals help in balancing both Pitta and the increasing Vata.
  - Soups, steamed veggies, and warm grain dishes are preferable.

2. Opt for Sweet, Bitter, and Astringent Tastes:
  - Sweet flavours cool down the heated Pitta without aggravating Vata (e.g., sweet fruits like grapes, pears, and apples).

- Bitter and astringent foods help detoxify any excess Pitta accumulated over the summer. Include foods like kale, spinach, brussels sprouts, and cranberries.

3. Reduce Pungent, Salty, and Sour Tastes:
- These tastes can aggravate Pitta. Limit foods like chili peppers, sour fruits, and very salty snacks.

4. Incorporate Cooling Herb and Spices:
- While moderate use of spices is good to stimulate digestion, prioritize cooling spices such as fennel, coriander, cardamom, and mint. These helps soothe excess Pitta without dampening digestive fire.
- Turmeric and cumin are also beneficial—they aid digestion and have anti-inflammatory properties.

5. Ensure Adequate Hydration:
- Continue to drink plenty of fluids but opt for room temperature or warm drinks instead of cold ones. Herbal teas like chamomile, dandelion, or liquorice root tea can be beneficial.

6. Dairy and Oils:
- Moderate amounts of dairy products can be soothing for Pitta. Choose options like ghee, milk, and soft cheeses.
- Cooling oils like coconut and olive oil are excellent for cooking and dressings.

Lifestyle Tips for Autumn:
- Daily Routine: Try to follow a regular daily routine to pacify the mobile quality of Vata.

- Skin Care: Moisturize regularly to protect the skin against the drying effects of the cooler, windy weather.
- Exercise: Opt for moderate exercises that do not overheat the body, such as swimming, walking, or yoga.

By adjusting your diet and lifestyle according to these guidelines, you can help manage Pitta during its late flare-up and transition smoothly into the cooler Vata-dominated season. Balancing these doshas promotes overall health, vitality, and well-being in the face of seasonal changes.

B. **Preparing for the Cold – Autumn Detox**

Preparing for the cooling months of autumn and upcoming winter involves helping the body adjust and align with the changing environment. Autumn is a pivotal time for detoxification or cleansing, especially as we transition from a potentially Pitta-aggravating summer into a Vata-dominant winter. This detoxification is critical for clearing Pitta accumulation and preventing Vata imbalance as the climate becomes drier and colder. The process includes dietary modifications, lifestyle adjustments, and specific Ayurvedic practices.

1. Dietary Adjustments for Autumn Detox

- Favor Warm, Cooked Foods: As the weather cools, include more warm, nourishing foods such as soups, stews, and cooked grains. These foods are easier to digest and help maintain internal warmth.

- Incorporate Spices: Utilize spices like turmeric, cumin, coriander, fennel, and ginger. These not only enhance digestion but also have cleansing properties which help in eliminating toxins.

- Reduce Heavy Foods: Cut down on dairy products, meats, and oils, as these can be heavy and aggravate Kapha when eaten in excess. Focus instead on lighter proteins like legumes and lentils.

- Include Bitter and Astringent Foods: Foods with these tastes help in purifying the blood and eliminating toxins. Examples include bitter greens (kale, spinach), barley, and apples.

- Stay Hydrated: Continue to drink plenty of fluids, opting for warm beverages like herbal teas which promote digestion and warmth. Ginger tea or cumin-coriander-fennel tea are excellent choices.

2. Ayurvedic Practices for Autumn Detox

- Panchakarma: Consider undergoing Panchakarma, a series of Ayurvedic detoxification treatments, under the supervision of an experienced practitioner. This can include procedures like Virechana (purification) and Basti (enema) tailored to individual needs.

- Daily Oil Massage (Abhyanga): Regularly massaging the body with warm sesame oil can help mitigate increased Vata, improving circulation and calming the nervous system.

- Steam Bath (Swedana): Following Abhyanga, a gentle steam bath can help open body channels and facilitate the removal of impurities via the skin.

- Nasya: Administer oil into the nostrils to cleanse accumulated Kapha and protect the respiratory passages from the dry and cold air.

3. Lifestyle Adjustments for Autumn

- Regular Exercise: Engage in regular but gentle exercise to boost circulation and aid detoxification. Yoga and walking are ideal as they are also grounding and help balance Vata.

- Sleep Adequately: Ensure to get enough rest as the nights grow longer, aiming for bed before 10 p.m. and rising with the sun to support natural circadian rhythms.

- Embrace Warmth: Keep warm with appropriate clothing to prevent Vata from becoming aggravated by the cold.

- Mental Detox: Include practices such as meditation or pranayama (breathing exercises) to support mental clarity and tranquillity, reducing stress which can exacerbate Vata.

An autumn detox centres on adjusting to the cooler, windier conditions by nurturing the body and preparing it physically and mentally. This involves cleaning up the diet, incorporating specific Ayurvedic practices, and making lifestyle tweaks that all aim to balance Pitta and ward off Vata's cold and erratic influence. Through these practices, one can enhance vitality and immunity, paving the way for a healthy winter season.

C. <u>Autumn-Specific Asanas and Exercise Routines</u>

As the seasons transition from the heat of summer to the cooler, windier days of autumn, the Pitta dosha that likely accumulated during the warmer months may still be high. Tailoring your yoga practice and exercise routines to address this imbalance can help you harmonize your internal environment with the shifting external climate. The focus in autumn should be on calming any residual heat in the body while beginning to counteract the dry and light qualities of increasing Vata.

Autumn-Specific Yoga Asanas
To balance aggravated Pitta and prepare for rising Vata, include asanas that are cooling and grounding, yet stabilizing and strengthening. These poses will help soothe Pitta while also addressing the mobile and erratic nature of Vata.

1. Moon Salutations (Chandra Namaskara)
   - Unlike Sun Salutations, Moon Salutations are cooling and soothing, making them perfect for

balancing Pitta. They include circular, flowing movements that are gentle and meditative, helping to calm the mind and body.

2. Seated Forward Bend (Paschimottanasana)
   - Forward bends are excellent for cooling the body and calming the brain, making them beneficial for reducing Pitta. They also increase the Vata-balancing qualities of grounding and introspection.

3. Camel Pose (Ustrasana)
   - This gentle backbend opens up the chest and lungs, counteracting the tendency of Pitta to accumulate in these areas. It also stimulates abdominal organs, aiding digestion—a common site of Pitta issues.

4. Tree Pose (Vrikshasana)
   - A balancing pose that fosters both physical and emotional stability, which is crucial for calming Vata and maintaining focus and calm as Pitta is balanced.

5. Marichi's Pose (Marichyasana)
   - This seated twist is excellent for massaging the abdominal organs, thereby improving digestion and elimination, which can be problematic in Pitta types. It's also soothing and grounding.

Cooling Pranayama Techniques
Breathing exercises can significantly influence our internal temperature and mental state. Incorporating cooling pranayama techniques can help in reducing Pitta:

1. Sheetali Pranayama (Cooling Breath)
   - This involves inhaling through a curled tongue to cool the body and calm the mind, perfect for excess Pitta.

2. Nadi Shodhana (Alternate Nostril Breathing)
   - This technique balances the body and mind by harmonizing the left and right hemispheres of the brain, reducing both Pitta and Vata.

Exercise Routines
Autumn is a good time to start integrating more grounding and stabilizing exercises into your routine:

1. Walking
   - Regular walks, particularly in natural, serene settings, can be incredibly grounding and are excellent for mental well-being.

2. Moderate Cycling
   - Engaging in a gentle cycling session, particularly during the cooler parts of the day, can be invigorating without aggravating Pitta.

3. Swimming
   - If accessible, swimming in natural, cool waters can be refreshingly calming and a great workout for the whole body without increasing heat.

Dietary Considerations
Complement your physical activities and asanas with a Pitta-pacifying diet. Favor cool, refreshing foods and those with a sweet, bitter, or astringent taste. Avoid

spicy, fermented, and sour foods which increase Pitta. Increase intake of dairy products, grains, and sweet fruits and vegetables.

By emphasizing cooling and grounding practices in your yoga and daily routines, you can effectively manage the transition through autumn, balancing Pitta, and preparing the body and mind for the eventual dominance of Vata as the season progresses.

D. **<u>Recipes for Autumn – Calming Pitta</u>**

Autumn, depending on the region, can still exhibit remnants of summer heat, particularly in the early weeks, which may aggravate Pitta dosha, characterized by qualities of heat and intensity. Shifting your diet to include foods that are cooling, grounding, and hydrating can help in soothing Pitta imbalance. Below are several recipes designed to calm Pitta during the autumn transition, incorporating sweet, bitter, and astringent tastes that are beneficial during this season.

1. Coconut Cucumber Soup
Ingredients:
- 1 large cucumber, peeled and chopped
- 1 can coconut milk
- 2 cups vegetable broth
- 1 tbsp lemon juice
- 1 tbsp fresh mint, chopped
- Salt and white pepper, to taste

Instructions:

1. In a blender, puree the cucumber with coconut milk until smooth.
2. Transfer the mixture to a pot and add the vegetable broth. Heat over medium heat but do not boil.
3. Just before serving, stir in lemon juice and mint. Season with salt and white pepper.
4. Serve chilled for additional cooling effects.

This soup is cooling, making it ideal for balancing Pitta. The cucumber and coconut milk are both hydrating and soothing.

2. Quinoa Salad with Pomegranate and Mint
Ingredients:
- 1 cup quinoa, cooked and cooled
- 1 pomegranate, seeded
- ½ cup chopped cucumber
- ¼ cup chopped fresh mint
- 2 tbsp olive oil
- Juice of 1 lemon
- Salt and black pepper, to taste

Instructions:
1. In a large bowl, combine the cooked quinoa, pomegranate seeds, cucumber, and mint.
2. In a small bowl, whisk together the olive oil, lemon juice, salt, and pepper.
3. Pour the dressing over the quinoa mixture and toss to combine.
4. Refrigerate for at least one hour before serving to allow the flavours to meld.

Quinoa provides a high-protein yet light base, while pomegranate and mint add fresh, soothing flavours, perfect for reducing Pitta.

3. Baked Pears with Cinnamon and Honey
Ingredients:
- 4 ripe pears, halved and cored
- 2 tbsp honey
- ½ tsp ground cinnamon
- A pinch of nutmeg
- ¼ cup crushed walnuts (optional)

Instructions:
1. Preheat the oven to 350°F (175°C).
2. Place the pear halves on a baking dish, cut side up.
3. Drizzle honey over each pear half and sprinkle with cinnamon and nutmeg.
4. Bake in the preheated oven for about 20-25 minutes, or until the pears are soft and slightly caramelized.
5. Serve warm, topped with crushed walnuts if using.

Sweet and mildly spiced, these baked pears are not only a delicious dessert but also a great way to calm Pitta. The sweetness of the pears and honey together with the warmth of cinnamon provides a soothing effect.

4. Green Bean Almondine with Lemon
Ingredients:
- 1 lb fresh green beans, trimmed
- 1 tbsp olive oil
- ½ cup sliced almonds

- Juice of 1 lemon
- Salt and black pepper, to taste

Instructions:
1. Blanch the green beans in boiling water for 3-4 minutes until they are bright green and tender crisp. Drain and rinse under cold water to stop the cooking process.
2. Heat the olive oil in a skillet over medium heat. Add the almonds and toast them lightly, stirring frequently, until golden brown.
3. Add the blanched green beans and lemon juice to the skillet. Toss to combine and heat through.
4. Season with salt and black pepper. Serve warm.

This dish is light and refreshing, with the astringent and bitter taste of green beans complimented by the zesty lemon, making it ideal for balancing Pitta.

These recipes are crafted to aid in reducing Pitta dosha during autumn, focusing on fresh, hydrating, and gentle flavours that align well with the needs of the season. They can help manage the body's internal heat and ensure a smooth transition into the cooler months.

Chapter 5: Winter - Nourishment and Conservation

A. Overview of Winter Characteristics and Dietary Needs

Winter in Ayurveda is split into two phases, Hemant (early winter) and Shishir (late winter), each characterized by distinct climatic conditions and corresponding impacts on bodily doshas, specifically the increase in Vata and potential accumulation of Kapha. Addressing these changes through diet and lifestyle is crucial to maintain balance and health during these colder months.

Winter Characteristics

Hemant (Early Winter)
- **Climate:** This phase is marked by cold and dry weather. Despite the chill, there is often a sense of stability in the air.
- **Dosha Influence:** Vata is still prominent due to the cold and dryness, but Kapha begins to accumulate because of the colder temperatures slowing down bodily processes.

- **Health Impact:** People might experience increased dryness of the skin, hair, and mucous membranes, joint pain, and digestive issues due to heightened Vata. The cold may also begin to cause some sluggishness or lethargy as Kapha increases.

Shishir (Late Winter)
- **Climate:** Characterized by even colder and potentially wetter conditions as it transitions towards spring.
- **Dosha Influence:** Kapha becomes more dominant, building upon the earlier accumulation during early winter.
- **Health Impact:** Common issues include colds, congestion, and excess mucus, alongside increased lethargy and weight gain if Kapha is not balanced.

Dietary Needs for Winter
The key to balancing health in winter lies in nurturing and warming the body while keeping Vata calm and preventing Kapha from accumulating excessively. Here are dietary considerations for each phase:

Hemant (Early Winter)
- **Warm, Nourishing Foods:** Focus on hearty, warming foods like soups, stews, and casseroles. Utilize healthy fats and oils, which are beneficial for combating the dryness associated with increased Vata.
- **Spices:** Incorporate warming spices such as ginger, garlic, cinnamon, cloves, cardamom, and black pepper to stimulate digestion and heat the body internally.
- **Proteins:** Increased intake of proteins is advised to build and maintain strength. Good sources include

legumes, nuts, seeds, and for non-vegetarians, eggs, and meats.
- **Root Vegetables:** Foods like carrots, potatoes, beets, and onions are grounding and provide sustained energy, which helps balance Vata.

Shishir (Late Winter)
- **Slightly Lighter Foods:** As Kapha dominates, transitioning towards lighter fare can help. However, the food should still be warm and moderately oily to counteract the cold.
- **Grains:** Incorporate whole grains like oatmeal, quinoa, and barley which offer Fiber and help in maintaining good digestion without increasing Kapha significantly.
- **Dairy:** If tolerable, warm, spiced milk can be comforting. However, excessive dairy can increase Kapha, so it should be consumed in moderation.
- **Fruits:** Favor seasonal fruits that are not too sweet or heavy. Apples and pears are ideal as they are lighter and can be cooked for better digestibility.
- **Vegetables:** Favor astringent, bitter, and pungent vegetables like brussels sprouts, cabbage, and kale; these can help counterbalance the heavy quality of Kapha.

General Winter Diet Tips
- **Stay Hydrated:** Despite the less intense thirst in winter, maintaining hydration is crucial. Warm drinks like herbal teas or warm water can aid digestion and warmth.

- **Eat Regularly:** Have meals at regular times to create a routine, which helps in managing Vata's irregular nature.
- **Avoid Cold Foods:** Ice creams, cold drinks, or excessively raw foods can aggravate Vata and hinder the digestive fire, which is already slower in cold conditions.

Addressing the dual challenges of Vata and Kapha in winter through a thoughtful diet is essential in Ayurveda. By adjusting food choices and cooking styles seasonally, one can effectively support their body's needs, promoting health and well-being throughout the colder months.

B. Strengthening Immunity in Winter

Winter is a season that naturally prompts the body to conserve energy and build strength to combat the cold and flu season, characterized by increased Kapha and Vata doshas. Strengthening immunity during this time is vital in Ayurveda and involves holistic practices that enhance both physical health and emotional well-being. Here are several Ayurvedic strategies to boost immunity during the winter months:

1. Dietary Adjustments
Warm, Cooked Foods: During winter, the digestive system can handle richer foods due to a stronger digestive fire (Agni). Opt for warm, nourishing foods like soups, stews, and curries that are cooked with immune-boosting spices such as turmeric, ginger, cumin, black pepper, and garlic.

Seasonal Fruits and Vegetables: Incorporate seasonal produce that is high in vitamins and antioxidants. Root vegetables (like carrots, beets, and turnips) and winter greens (such as kale, spinach, and Swiss chard) are excellent. Fruits like oranges, pomegranates, and apples offer vitamin C, which is crucial for immune function.

Herbs and Spices: Herbs like Ashwagandha, Tulsi (Holy Basil), and spices like turmeric have immune-modulating properties and can help the body resist stress, a key factor in immune health.

2. Regular Physical Activity

Maintaining a regular exercise routine is crucial in winter to keep the lymphatic system flowing, which helps remove toxins from the body and increases the efficiency of the immune system. Yoga, brisk walking, and light jogging are good options that do not exhaust the body but keep it active and warmed up.

3. Adequate Sleep

Good quality sleep is a cornerstone of good health and immune function. The body repairs and regenerates tissues during sleep, and important immune-boosting compounds are released. Aim for 7-9 hours of sleep per night and try to maintain a consistent sleep schedule.

4. Manage Stress

Chronic stress can suppress the immune system and make you more vulnerable to illness. Incorporate stress-reduction techniques such as meditation, yoga, deep breathing exercises, and mindful relaxation. Practices like Yoga Nidra and Abhyanga (self-massage with warm oil) are especially beneficial for balancing Vata and reducing stress.

5. Stay Hydrated

Although you might not feel as thirsty during winter, maintaining adequate hydration is crucial for optimal immune function. Warm teas and hot water infused with immune-supportive herbs like ginger, cinnamon, or licorice root can be both hydrating and warming.

6. Pranayama (Breathwork)

Specific pranayama techniques such as Anulom Vilom (Alternate Nostril Breathing) and Kapalbhati (Skull Shining Breath) can help maintain heat in the body and clear the channels of circulation, potentially boosting resistance to colds and other respiratory illnesses.

7. Ayurvedic Supplements

Consider supplements like Chyawanprash, a traditional Ayurvedic herbal tonic that is renowned for its immune-enhancing properties. It contains Amalaki (Indian gooseberry) as a primary ingredient, rich in Vitamin C, along with over 40 other natural herbs and spices that support immune health, digestion, and overall vitality.

8. Seasonal Cleansing

Winter is a good time for gentle cleansing to reset the digestive system and eliminate toxins (Ama) that could impair the immune system. A simple Kitchari cleanse (eating a diet of mainly Kitchari — a dish of mung beans and rice seasoned with spices — for several days) can be effective.

By integrating these Ayurvedic principles and practices into your winter routine, you can effectively boost your body's defenses and maintain your health during the colder months.

C. Winter-Specific Asanas and Warm Therapies

During the cold months of winter, maintaining internal warmth and circulation becomes crucial not only for comfort but also for preventing the aggravation of Vata dosha, which tends to increase with cold and dry conditions. Yoga practices and warm therapies can be especially beneficial to stimulate circulation, support the immune system, and help the body and mind stay balanced and energized. Here are some winter-specific asanas and warm therapies recommended in Ayurveda.

Winter-Specific Asanas
1. Sun Salutations (Surya Namaskar)
   - This sequence warms up the whole body, stretches all the major muscles, boosts circulation, and is an excellent way to maintain flexibility and strength during winter.

2. Warrior Poses (Virabhadrasana I & II)
  - These poses are energizing, improve balance and stability, enhance circulation, and warm up the body effectively.

3. Chair Pose (Utkatasana)
  - A heat-generating pose that strengthens the lower back, thighs, and calves while stimulating the heart and diaphragm.

4. Twists (like Ardha Matsyendrasana - Half Lord of the Fishes Pose)
  - Twists are great for maintaining digestive fire, which is crucial for maintaining strong immunity and efficient metabolism during colder months.

5. Backbends (such as Bhujangasana - Cobra Pose, or Ustrasana - Camel Pose)
  - Gentle backbends warm the spine and heart, promoting better circulation and respiratory health.

6. Inversion poses (like Legs-Up-The-Wall Pose - Viparita Karani)
  - These help in venous return (blood flow back to the heart), are calming for the nervous system, and are warming from the inside out.

Warm Therapies
1. Abhyanga (Self-Massage with Warm Oil)
  - A traditional Ayurvedic technique that involves massaging the body with ample amounts of warm sesame oil (or other Vata-pacifying oils like almond or olive oil). This not only nourishes and soothes dry

skin but also increases circulation and calms the nervous system.

2. Steam Therapy (Swedana)
   - Following oil massage, sitting in a steam room or taking a warm bath can help the body further relax and detoxify. The warmth helps open up the pores, allowing the oil to penetrate deeper and toxins to exit.

3. Sipping Warm Herbal Teas
   - Drinking teas made with ginger, cinnamon, cardamom, or cloves throughout the day keeps the body warm and aids digestion.

4. Warm Packs
   - Applying warm packs on tense areas like the neck, shoulders, or lower back can relieve stiffness and pain, which may worsen in cold weather due to increased Vata.

5. Heated Yoga
   - Practicing yoga in a slightly warmer environment can be beneficial during the winter. If you don't have access to a heated yoga studio, ensuring your practice space is warm enough can also help.

6. Ginger Baths
   - Adding powdered ginger to a warm bath can stimulate body warmth and circulation, acting as a whole-body warming agent.

7. Warm Foot Baths

- Soaking feet in warm water before bedtime can improve circulation and help in relaxing and getting a good night's sleep.

Implementing these asanas and warm therapies during the winter season will help sustain your body's inner heat, enhance blood flow, reduce muscle stiffness, and ward off the cold, providing a robust defense against the increase in Vata. Additionally, these practices support robust health by promoting better digestion, immunity, and overall vitality during the colder months.

D. Recipes for Winter – Nourishing and Heating Foods

Winter calls for nourishment and warmth from within, especially as Vata dosha can become aggravated due to the cold and dry weather, leading to issues like dry skin, discomfort in joints, and digestive problems. Here are some Ayurvedic-inspired recipes tailored for winter to provide warmth, hydration, and balance.

1. Spiced Lentil Soup
Ingredients:
- 1 cup red lentils, rinsed and drained
- 1 onion, finely chopped
- 2 garlic cloves, minced
- 2 carrots, diced
- 1 celery stalk, diced
- 1 teaspoon turmeric powder
- 1 teaspoon cumin seeds

- 1/2 teaspoon ground coriander
- 1/2 teaspoon ground ginger
- 6 cups vegetable broth or water
- 2 tablespoons olive oil or ghee
- Salt and pepper, to taste
- Fresh cilantro or parsley, chopped for garnish

Instructions:
1. Heat the olive oil or ghee in a large pot over medium heat. Add the cumin seeds and wait until they start to sputter.
2. Add the onions, garlic, carrots, and celery, and sauté until the onions are translucent.
3. Stir in turmeric, coriander, and ginger, cooking for another minute.
4. Add the lentils and vegetable broth. Bring to a boil, then lower the heat and simmer covered for about 25-30 minutes, or until the lentils are soft.
5. Season with salt and pepper. Serve hot, garnished with fresh cilantro or parsley.

This soup is warming and grounding, perfect for balancing Vata. The spices used are great for stimulating digestion, essential in the cold months.

2. Warming Oatmeal with Spiced Apples

Ingredients for Oatmeal:
- 1 cup rolled oats
- 2 cups water or milk
- A pinch of salt

Ingredients for Spiced Apples:
- 1 apple, peeled and chopped
- 1/2 teaspoon ground cinnamon
- 1/4 teaspoon ground nutmeg
- 1 tablespoon ghee
- 1 tablespoon maple syrup or honey

Instructions:
1. In a saucepan, bring the water or milk to a boil. Add oats and salt, reduce heat, and simmer, stirring occasionally until the oats are cooked, about 10-15 minutes.
2. For the spiced apples, melt ghee in a skillet over medium heat. Add the chopped apples, cinnamon, and nutmeg. Cook until the apples are soft and fragrant. Stir in maple syrup or honey.
3. Serve the warm oatmeal topped with spiced apples.

This breakfast is ideal for warming up on a cold winter morning, providing sustained energy and aiding digestion with its beneficial spices.

3. Ginger Turmeric Tea
Ingredients:
- 1-inch fresh ginger root, thinly sliced
- 1/2-inch fresh turmeric root, thinly sliced (or 1 teaspoon turmeric powder)
- 4 cups water
- Honey to taste (optional)
- Lemon juice to taste (optional)

Instructions:

1. In a saucepan, bring water to a boil. Add sliced ginger and turmeric.
2. Reduce the heat and simmer for about 10-15 minutes.
3. Strain the tea into cups. Add honey and lemon juice to taste if desired.

This tea is excellent for warming the body, boosting circulation, and supporting the immune system during the winter months. Ginger and turmeric both have anti-inflammatory properties and are known for their warming effects.

4. Roasted Root Vegetables

Ingredients:
- A mix of root vegetables (carrots, parsnips, sweet potatoes, beets), peeled and cubed
- 2 tablespoons olive oil or ghee
- 1 teaspoon rosemary, chopped
- Salt and pepper, to taste

Instructions:
1. Preheat the oven to 400°F (200°C).
2. Toss the cubed vegetables with olive oil or ghee, rosemary, salt, and pepper.
3. Spread the vegetables on a baking sheet in a single layer.
4. Roast in the oven for about 40 minutes, stirring halfway through, until vegetables are tender and caramelized.

Roasted root vegetables are grounding, nourishing, and provide essential fibers and vitamins, helping to keep Vata in balance.

These recipes not only provide warmth and nourishment but also help maintain balance in the doshas during the winter months, ensuring comfort and promoting health.

Chapter 6: Transitioning Between Seasons

A. Recognizing the Subtle Changes

Transitioning between seasons is a delicate time for the body as it adjusts to changing environmental conditions. According to Ayurveda, each season brings unique qualities that influence the three doshas—Vata, Pitta, and Kapha. Recognizing subtle changes in your body and environment is key to adapting your lifestyle and maintaining balance. Here's how you can better understand and manage these transitions effectively:

1. Observing Environmental Changes
One of the first steps in adjusting to a new season is to become more attentive to environmental alterations:

- Temperature: Shifts in temperature are clear indicators of a changing season. Cooling temperatures signal a move from summer to autumn, while warming trends indicate a transition from winter to spring.

- Humidity and Dryness: Notice the moisture level in the air. Humidity often increases as we move into summer and decreases entering autumn and winter, impacting your internal dosha balance.

- Wind and Weather Patterns: Increased wind can suggest a transition towards or within autumn, prominently increasing Vata. Conversely, calming winds might indicate a shift towards summer, where Pitta can become predominant.

- Daylight: The length of the day and the intensity of sunlight directly affect your dosha balance and physical and psychological well-being.

2. Noticing Physical Responses
Your body reacts to environmental changes, often manifesting symptoms that correspond to shifts in dosha balance:

- Energy Levels: An upsurge or reduction in energy levels can indicate doshic shifts. For example, increased lethargy during early spring can suggest an accumulation of Kapha.

- Appetite and Digestion: Changes in appetite or digestive strength often occur with seasonal shifts. For instance, a stronger appetite in winter is a natural response to increased Agni (digestive fire), while a sluggish digestion in spring suggests heightened Kapha.

- Skin and Hair Condition: Dry or oily skin and hair can indicate how environmental changes are impacting your Vata or Kapha dosha. For example, dry, rough, and cracked skin often accompanies an increase in Vata during autumn.

3. Emotional and Mental Changes

Seasonal transitions can also influence your emotional and mental states:

- Mood Fluctuations: You might experience mood swings as the seasons change. For instance, the decrease in sunlight during autumn and winter can lead to feelings of sadness or depression.

- Stress Levels: Varying stress levels can be a sign of struggling to adapt to new seasonal patterns, impacting your overall dosha balance.

4. Sleep Patterns

Changes in sleep patterns provide clues to how well your body is adapting to new seasonal influences:

- Sleep Quality and Duration: An increase in sleep disturbances or a change in your sleep requirements can reflect an imbalance in doshas. Increased sleep during winter might indicate an excess of Kapha, while disturbed sleep during autumn might suggest elevated Vata.

Practical Tips for Managing Seasonal Transitions

- Diet: Adjust your diet according to the season. Lighter, cooler foods in summer help pacify Pitta, while warmer, oily, and heavier foods in winter balance Vata.
- Routine: Maintain a consistent daily routine suitable for the upcoming season. Adjust sleeping and eating times to align more closely with natural light patterns.
- Exercise: Adapt your physical activities to support the dominant seasonal dosha. Energizing activities are suitable for spring and calming ones for autumn.
- Preventative Detox: Engaging in a seasonal detox (such as Panchakarma) can help reset your digestive system and clear accumulated doshas from the previous season.

By tuning into these subtle shifts, you can make conscious decisions to align your lifestyle with the natural rhythms of the environment, enhancing your health and well-being throughout each seasonal transition.

B. Adjusting Diet and Practices During Seasonal Shifts

Adjusting your diet and daily practices to align with seasonal shifts is a central tenet of Ayurveda. As each season affects the balance of the doshas (Vata, Pitta, and Kapha), altering your routines can help maintain equilibrium in your body and mind. Here's how to adapt your diet and lifestyle practices during these transitions:

1. Transition from Winter to Spring:

- Diet: Focus on gradually reducing heavy and oily foods characteristic of winter diets. Introduce more bitter, astringent, and pungent flavors which help to cleanse accumulated Kapha. Include leafy greens, sprouts, and seeds.
- Practices: Increase physical activity to shake off the winter sluggishness. Spring is a good time for detoxification, so consider lighter meals and perhaps a structured cleanse like a Kitchari cleanse. Begin to wake up a bit earlier and enjoy the increasing hours of daylight.

2. Transition from Spring to Summer:
- Diet: Shift towards cooling and lighter foods to balance the increasing Pitta. Favor sweet, bitter, and astringent tastes. Include fruits such as watermelon, berries, and apples, and vegetables like cucumbers, leafy greens, and zucchini.
- Practices: Engage in cooling activities, such as swimming or moonlit walks. Practice cooling pranayama techniques like Sheetali or Sheetkari. Start your day earlier to avoid the midday heat, which is when Pitta is at its peak.

3. Transition from Summer to Autumn:
- Diet: As the heat dissipates, begin incorporating warm, grounding foods to pacify Vata. Increase your intake of root vegetables, nuts, whole grains, and oils. Warm spices such as ginger, cinnamon, and cloves can be revitalizing.
- Practices: Introduce grounding yoga practices and stabilize energy through routines such as regular mealtimes and earlier bedtime hours. This period is

critical for nourishing the body in preparation for winter.

4. Transition from Autumn to Winter:
- Diet: With the onset of colder weather, the diet should become more nourishing and richer. Incorporate hearty soups, stews, and roasted root vegetables. Foods should be well-spiced to keep the digestive fire burning, using black pepper, fenugreek, mustard seeds, and asafoetida.
- Practices: Focus on indoor, warming exercises like hot yoga or strength training to keep the body active despite the cold. Ensure your home environment is warm and cozy and consider practices like warm oil massages (Abhyanga) to keep skin nourished and circulation active.

General Tips:
- Stay Hydrated: Regardless of the season, maintaining adequate hydration is crucial. Modify the temperature of the water you drink according to the season – warm in winter and cool (not cold) in summer.
- Adjust Sleep Patterns: Go to bed earlier in winter to conserve energy and slightly later in summer to enjoy the longer days, always aiming for 7-9 hours of restful sleep.
- Mindfulness and Meditation: Regular mindfulness practice can help you stay connected to your body's needs and the subtle changes in your environment.

Herbal Support:

- Winter to Spring: Use warming herbs like ginger and black pepper to kickstart the digestive fire that might be sluggish from winter.
- Spring to Summer: Incorporate cooling herbs such as fennel, coriander, and mint to soothe excess heat.
- Summer to Autumn: Transition with grounding herbs like ashwagandha which stabilizes both mind and body.
- Autumn to Winter: Use tonifying herbs such as tulsi and ginseng to build internal strength and immunity.

By being attentive to the needs of your body and adjusting your diet and practices with the seasonal shifts, you can enhance your health, vitality, and well-being throughout the year.

C. Tips for Smooth Transition

Transitioning smoothly between seasons, or during any period of change, requires a mindful approach that aligns with both the internal state of your body and the external environment. Ayurveda, through its concept of Ritusandhi, emphasizes practical and effective ways to navigate these shifts. Here are tips for ensuring a smooth transition:

1. Gradual Dietary Shifts
Adjust your diet progressively. As one season fades into the next, start incorporating elements of the upcoming season's diet while phasing out foods from the current season. For instance:

- Winter to Spring: Reduce heavy, oily foods and dairy a few weeks before spring and introduce lighter meals that are easier to digest.
- Summer to Autumn: Start reducing very cold, raw foods and increase warm, cooked meals.

2. Monitor Agni (Digestive Fire)

Seasonal changes often impact your digestive strength. Maintain a strong Agni by:
- Eating at regular times and avoiding snacking between meals.
- Using spices appropriate for the upcoming season—like ginger and cinnamon in winter for their warming properties.

3. Adapt Your Exercise Routine

Adjust your physical activity according to the season:
- Spring: Increase vigorous activities to shed winter weight and boost circulation.
- Summer: Opt for cooling exercises like swimming or early morning yoga to avoid overheating.
- Autumn and Winter: Incorporate more grounding and strengthening exercises, like weight training or indoor aerobic exercises to keep warm and stable.

4. Hydration

Adapt your hydration habits to reflect seasonal needs:
- In summer, increase intake of cooling drinks and watery fruits.

- In winter, opt for warm beverages like herbal teas to maintain internal warmth and hydration.

5. Mindfulness and Mental Health

Each season can affect your mental and emotional health differently:
- Practice mindfulness and meditation regularly to reduce stress and adapt more easily to change.
- Engage in seasonal activities that promote mental well-being, such as nature walks in autumn or journaling in winter.

6. Sleep Adjustments

Sleep patterns can require adjustments to align with natural light variations:
- Go to bed earlier in winter to conserve energy.
- Stay active later into the evening in summer to enjoy the longer days.

7. Skin Care Adjustments

Your skin reacts to environmental changes, so adapt your skin care routine:
- Use more moisturizing products in winter.
- Switch to lighter lotions or aloe-based products in summer.

8. Herbal Support

Incorporate seasonal herbs that support transition:
- Use detoxifying herbs like neem or turmeric during spring.

- In autumn, adaptogenic herbs like ashwagandha can help the body manage stress and adjust to cooler temperatures.

9. Clothing and Environment
Adjust your living environment and clothing:

- Transition your wardrobe gradually—layering is key during periods of fluctuating temperatures.
- Modify your home environment to maintain comfort, such as using humidifiers in dry winter months or fans and light drapes in summer.

10. Regular Cleansing
Consider seasonal detoxification practices to clear accumulated doshas and refresh the system, particularly at the junction between seasons:
- Conduct a simple Ayurvedic cleanse at home with a mono-diet of kitchari (a nourishing mix of rice and mung beans) for a few days.
- Visit an Ayurvedic practitioner for personalized detoxifying procedures like Panchakarma.

Adapting these practices into your routines during transition periods will help you maintain stability and health throughout each seasonal shift, allowing your body and mind to acclimate naturally and efficiently.

Chapter 7: Mind and Mood: Seasonal Impacts on Mental Health

A. Seasonal Affective Disorder in Ayurveda

Seasonal Affective Disorder (SAD) is a type of depression that typically occurs during the autumn and winter months when daylight hours are shorter. In Ayurveda, while not explicitly termed as "Seasonal Affective Disorder," similar conditions are understood through the lens of doshic imbalances and changes in natural rhythms that affect the mind and body. The winter season is generally dominated by the Vata dosha, which embodies qualities of movement, dryness, and coldness, and if aggravated, can lead to mental health disturbances including anxiety and depressive symptoms.

Understanding SAD in Ayurveda:

In Ayurvedic terms, the cold, dry, and often erratic energy of Vata can disturb the nervous system, leading to feelings of anxiety, loneliness, sadness, and lethargy — all symptoms commonly associated with SAD. The lack of sunlight contributes to disruptions in serotonin and melatonin levels, which are crucial regulators of mood, sleep, and appetite, further compounding these Vata imbalances.

Ayurvedic Management of SAD:

1. Diet Adjustments:

- Nourishing Foods: Increase the intake of warm, oily, and grounding foods that balance Vata. This includes foods like root vegetables, whole grains, nuts, and seeds, along with healthy fats like ghee and olive oil.

- Spices: Incorporate warming spices such as ginger, turmeric, cinnamon, and cloves to enhance digestion and circulation, both of which can have uplifting effects on your mood.

- Regular Meals: Eating meals at regular times helps to regulate the digestive fire (Agni) which is essential for optimal mental and physical health.

2. Lifestyle Changes:

- Light Exposure: Maximize exposure to natural light. Spend time outdoors during daylight hours and consider using a light therapy box that mimics natural sunlight.

- Routine: Establish a regular, soothing daily routine. Waking up, eating meals, and going to sleep at the

same times every day can help stabilize the body's internal clock.
- Physical Activity: Engage in regular physical activity like yoga, walking, or any exercise that helps reduce stress and anxiety. Yoga poses that are particularly grounding and pacifying for Vata include Tadasana (Mountain Pose), Balasana (Child's Pose), and Supta Baddha Konasana (Reclining Bound Angle Pose).

3. Herbal Remedies:
- Adaptogens: Herbs like Ashwagandha and Brahmi can be very helpful. Ashwagandha helps in combatting stress and boosting resilience, while Brahmi (Bacopa) is well-known for its cognitive-enhancing and mood-stabilizing properties. Also herbs like Tagar, Jatamansi and Yastimadhu can be used.
- Teas: Drinking herbal teas with Vata-balancing herbs like licorice, cinnamon, or tulsi can be comforting and soothing.

4. Mind-Body Therapies:
- Meditation and Pranayama: Practices such as guided meditation, mindfulness, and breathing exercises like Nadi Shodhana (Alternate Nostril Breathing) can be incredibly beneficial in managing stress and anxiety.
- Massage: Regular self-massage (Abhyanga) with warm oil (like sesame oil) can nourish the skin, soothe the nervous system, and support overall emotional well-being.

5. Social Interaction:
- Even when it's tempting to withdraw, maintaining social contact is vital. Regular interaction with friends and family, whether in-person or virtually, can provide significant emotional support.

6. Professional Guidance:
- It's important to work with a healthcare provider or an Ayurvedic practitioner to tailor these recommendations specifically for you, especially if symptoms are severe.

By addressing the physical, mental, and emotional aspects of health through these Ayurvedic practices, individuals prone to seasonal affective disorder can find relief and maintain a more balanced state throughout the changing seasons.

B. Mindful Practices for Emotional Stability

Achieving emotional stability is crucial for overall well-being and can be effectively supported by incorporating mindful practices into your daily routine. Mindfulness in the Ayurvedic context not only pertains to mental awareness but also involves harmonizing body, mind, and spirit to cultivate balance and tranquility. Here are various mindful practices that can foster emotional stability:

1. Daily Meditation

Consistent meditation is foundational for achieving emotional stability. It helps calm the mind, reduce stress, enhance self-awareness, and promote a state of peacefulness and clarity.

- Practice: Begin with just 5-10 minutes a day of seated meditation, focusing on your breath. Gradually increase the duration as you become more comfortable with the practice.
- Technique: Try mindfulness meditation where you observe your thoughts and feelings without judgment, letting them pass without getting attached to them.

2. Pranayama (Breath Control)
Pranayama, or breath control, directly influences the mind and can help in managing emotions effectively. Certain breathing techniques are especially helpful in cultivating emotional balance.

- Anulom Vilom (Alternate Nostril Breathing): This technique is excellent for balancing the left and right hemispheres of the brain, harmonizing emotional and logical aspects of the personality.
- Bhramari Pranayama (Bee Breath): Known for its immediate calming effects, this practice involves making a humming sound that vibrates in the head, soothing the nervous system.

3. Yoga Asanas

Physical postures in yoga not only improve body strength and flexibility but also help stabilize mood by reducing anxiety and stress levels.

- Balasana (Child's Pose): This is a resting pose that promotes feelings of safety and comfort, excellent for moments of emotional overwhelm.
- Setu Bandhasana (Bridge Pose): Helps open the chest, heart, and shoulders, areas where emotional tension is often held.

4. Mindful Eating

This practice involves paying full attention to the process of eating, focusing on the taste, texture, and aroma of your food, which aids in digesting both your food and emotions more effectively.

- Technique: Eat slowly and without distractions like TV or smartphones. Acknowledge the sources of your food and its potential effects on your body, cultivating gratitude for the nourishment it provides.

5. Nature Walks

Spending time in nature can significantly boost your mood and offer a new perspective, helping to ground your emotions.

- Practice: Engage in regular walks in natural settings. Be fully present, observing the sights, sounds, and smells around you without any rush.

6. Gratitude Journaling

Keeping a gratitude journal where you regularly write down things you are thankful for can shift your focus from negative to positive aspects of life, enhancing emotional resilience.

- Routine: Every night, write down three things you were grateful for that day. This practice can transform your mindset over time and is particularly powerful during challenging periods.

7. Art and Creative Expression
Engaging in creative activities such as drawing, painting, writing, or playing music allows emotional expression in a constructive and often therapeutic manner.

- Activity: Dedicate time each week to a creative hobby that relaxes you and allows you to express your feelings freely.

8. Counseling or Therapy
Sometimes, guided help from a professional can provide the tools and space needed to process emotions mindfully.

- Consideration: Regular sessions with a therapist can be powerful, especially when combined with Ayurvedic practices or other holistic approaches.

Incorporating these mindful practices into your lifestyle can help maintain emotional stability, providing a foundation of inner peace that supports overall health and well-being.

C. Meditation and Breathwork for Each Season

Meditation and breathwork (pranayama) are powerful tools in Ayurveda that can be tailored to align with the energetic qualities of each season. These practices help to harmonize body, mind, and spirit with the external environment, promoting health and well-being throughout the year.

1. Spring (Kapha Season)
Meditation Focus: Visualization and Decluttering
- Practice: Engage in meditation sessions that focus on clearing and rejuvenating the mind. Visualize fresh energy flowing into your life, as spring is a time of renewal.
- Technique: Imagine a clear stream washing away clutter, leaving behind clarity and freshness.

Breathwork: Kapalabhati (Skull Shining Breath)
- This stimulating breathing technique helps to clear mucus from the air passages, energize the mind, and reduce the heaviness associated with Kapha.
- How to Do It: Perform short, powerful exhales driven by the abdominal muscles, with passive inhales.

2. Summer (Pitta Season)
Meditation Focus: Cooling and Soothing

- Practice: Meditations that incorporate cooling imagery, such as a calm lake or moonlight, help to soothe Pitta's heat.
- Technique: Use guided imagery to visualize a serene, cool environment, feeling the coolness permeate your body.

Breathwork: Sheetali Pranayama (Cooling Breath)
- This breathwork cools the body and calms the mind, perfect for addressing Pitta's fiery nature.
- How to Do It: Curl the sides of your tongue upward and inhale through the mouth, hold for a moment, then exhale through the nose.

3. Autumn (Vata Season)

Meditation Focus: Grounding and Centering
- Practice: Since Vata is characterized by movement and change, focus your meditation on grounding. Visualization of roots growing from your body into the earth can be effective.
- Technique: Use a mantra such as "I am stable, I am grounded" to enhance the feeling of being centered and calm.

Breathwork: Nadi Shodhana (Alternate Nostril Breathing)
- This is a balancing breath that calms the mind, promotes focus, and stabilizes Vata.
- How to Do It: Gently close the right nostril with your right thumb, inhale through the left nostril, close it with your fingers, open the right nostril and

exhale. Repeat the process by inhaling through the right nostril.

4. Winter (Kapha/Vata Season)
Meditation Focus: Warmth and Light
- Practice: Meditations that center around inner warmth and light are beneficial during the cold, dark winter months.
- Technique: Visualize a warm, bright light at the heart center, spreading warmth and brightness throughout the body with each breath.

Breathwork: Bhastrika (Bellows Breath)
- This vigorous breathing practice heats the body and clears lethargy, countering the cold and stagnation of winter.
- How to Do It: Take quick, forceful breaths through the nose, actively engaging the diaphragm.

Tips for All Seasons
- Consistency: Aim to practice meditation and breathwork daily, ideally at the same time each day, to establish a routine that supports your body's circadian rhythm.
- Environment: Create a calm, inviting space for your practices. This might include elements like cushions, blankets, or subdued lighting.
- Preparation: Spend a few minutes settling into your practice. Begin by sitting comfortably, gently closing your eyes, and taking a few deep breaths to transition from the busyness of your day.

By adjusting your meditation themes and pranayama techniques with the seasons, you can better support your body's needs throughout the year, enhancing your overall health and well-being.

Chapter 8: Integrating Modern Life with Seasonal Ayurveda

A. Tips for Busy Lifestyles

In today's fast-paced world, integrating Ayurvedic principles into a busy lifestyle might seem challenging, yet it is entirely possible with some thoughtful planning and commitment. This chapter provides practical tips for incorporating seasonal Ayurveda into a hectic schedule, ensuring that even the busiest individuals can maintain balance and health throughout the year.

1. Plan and Prep Seasonal Meals
- Batch Cooking: Spend a couple of hours each week preparing and cooking large batches of seasonally appropriate meals that can be stored and eaten throughout the week. For instance, cook a big pot of

Kitchari in spring or a hearty vegetable stew in winter.

- Seasonal Foods List: Keep a list of seasonal foods on your fridge or phone. This makes grocery shopping quicker and ensures that you stick to an Ayurvedic diet suitable for the current season.

- Quick Recipes: Develop a repertoire of quick and easy recipes that align with Ayurvedic principles and can be whipped up in less than 30 minutes.

2. Regular Routines

- Dinacharya (Daily Routine): Even when time is scarce, maintain a simple version of the Ayurvedic daily routine. This includes waking up early, scraping your tongue, drinking warm water, and performing a short meditation or breathing exercises.

- Bedtime Routine: Aim to go to bed at the same time each night, which should ideally be before 10 PM to keep Pitta balanced. Wind down with a warm bath or gentle yoga to promote better sleep.

3. Seasonal Exercise Adjustments

- Efficient Workouts: Match your exercise to the season and your dosha. For instance, calming yoga or swimming in summer (Pitta season), and more vigorous activities like jogging or HIIT workouts in winter (Kapha season).

- Incorporate Exercise into Your Day: If finding a block of time is hard, break up your exercise into shorter, more manageable periods. For example, take a brisk 10-minute walk after each meal.

4. Mindful Practices
- Mobile Meditation: Use meditation apps for guided sessions that you can do anywhere, even during a lunch break or while commuting.
- Breathing Exercises: Utilize short pranayama practices throughout the day to stay balanced. Five minutes of Nadi Shodhana (Alternate Nostril Breathing) can be remarkably rejuvenating.

5. Leverage Technology
- Reminders: Set reminders on your phone for everything from drinking water to taking a deep breath, which can help maintain your Ayurvedic commitments.
- Apps and Resources: Use apps that track diet, menstrual cycles, exercise, and meditation to stay on top of your health with respect to Ayurvedic guidelines.

6. Seasonal Detox
- Simplified Cleanse: For those unable to perform traditional cleanses like Panchakarma due to time constraints, consider simpler detox methods such as a one-day juice cleanse or a weekend Ayurvedic detox involving light foods like kitchari.

7. Herbal and Natural Supplements
- Daily Supplements: Incorporate Ayurvedic herbs and supplements into your daily regime to support digestion, immunity, and overall well-being. Examples are Triphala for digestion or Ashwagandha for stress relief.

- Teas: Replace your afternoon coffee with herbal teas that fit the season — for instance, cooling peppermint in summer or invigorating ginger tea in winter.

8. Community and Support
- Support Group: Join or create a support group with like-minded individuals who are also trying to incorporate Ayurveda into their lives. Sharing tips, recipes, and successes can make the journey more enjoyable and less daunting.

By taking these adaptable and manageable steps, anyone can integrate the ancient wisdom of Ayurveda into the hustle and bustle of modern life, enhancing both physical health and mental clarity throughout the seasonal changes.

B. Quick Ayurvedic Hacks for Each Season

Incorporating Ayurvedic principles into your daily life doesn't need to be complex or time-consuming. Here are quick Ayurvedic hacks for each season to help align your body with the natural rhythms of the environment, ensuring optimal health year-round:

1. Spring (Kapha Season)
- Start the Day with Warm Water and Lemon: To stimulate digestion and remove toxins that accumulated during the colder months, drink a glass of warm water with lemon each morning.

- Dry Brushing: Before your shower, practice dry brushing your skin for about 5 minutes. This stimulates the lymphatic system, helping to remove Kapha accumulation in tissues.
- Incorporate Honey: Replace sugar with honey as a sweetener which is warming and aids in scraping excess Kapha from the channels.

2. Summer (Pitta Season)
- Coconut Oil Cooling: Apply coconut oil to your body before jumping into the shower. Coconut oil has cooling properties, perfect for soothing Pitta.
- Cucumber and Mint Water: Keep a jug of water infused with slices of cucumber and mint leaves in your refrigerator. This provides a deliciously cooling drink to pacify Pitta's heat.
- Rose Water Spritz: Keep a small spray bottle of rose water in your fridge and use it to spritz your face throughout the day for an immediate cooling effect.

3. Autumn (Vata Season)
- Warm Oil Massage: Each morning or before bed, give yourself a quick massage with warm sesame oil. This helps ground Vata's air and ether qualities.
- Spiced Milk: Before bed, drink warm milk boiled with spices like turmeric, ginger, and cardamom to soothe Vata and promote good sleep.
- Sweet, Sour, and Salty Foods: Integrate these tastes into your meals more frequently, as they balance Vata. Think cooked grains, soups, citrus fruits, and salted nuts.

4. Winter (Vata-Kapha Season)

- Ginger Tea: Start your day with a cup of warm ginger tea. This stimulates digestion and keeps the body warm and hydrated.
- Eat Root Vegetables: Incorporate more root vegetables like carrots, beets, and sweet potatoes into your diet. These are grounding and nourishing, helping to balance both Vata and Kapha.
- Warm, Spiced Breakfasts: Opt for warm cereals like cooked oatmeal or quinoa with cinnamon and cloves, which warm the interior of the body and combat the increased Vata and Kapha.

General Seasonal Tips

- Adjust Your Sleep: Go to bed earlier in winter (around 10 PM) and stay up a little later in summer (around 11 PM) to adapt to the natural light cycles and benefit your doshic balance.
- Flexible Exercise Routine: Tailor your physical activity based on the season — more invigorating and stimulating exercises in spring and summer, and more grounding, stabilizing activities in autumn and winter.

These simple, season-specific Ayurvedic hacks can easily be woven into your daily routine, allowing you to maintain harmony and health throughout the year.

C. Adapting Seasonal Ayurveda in Urban Settings

Adapting Ayurvedic principles to fit a modern, urban lifestyle can be a rewarding approach to maintaining health and wellness amidst the hustle and bustle of the city. Here are practical ways to integrate seasonal Ayurveda into your daily routine, even if you live in an urban setting:

1. Seasonal Diet Adaptation
- Local Farmers Markets: Even in urban areas, farmers markets are a valuable resource for fresh, locally grown produce. Make it a habit to visit them regularly to pick up seasonal fruits and vegetables which are crucial to Ayurvedic nutrition.
- Ayurvedic Meal Prepping: Dedicate a few hours each week to prepare seasonal dishes that align with Ayurvedic principles. Batch cooking can help you maintain a balanced diet during your busy week.

2. Mindful Practices Amidst City Life
- Morning Routine: Start your day with a brief session of yoga, meditation, or pranayama, which can be done even in small spaces. Establishing a calming morning routine can help set a positive tone for your day.
- Walking Meditation: Use your commute or daily walks as an opportunity for mindfulness. Pay attention to your breathing and stay present, which can be particularly grounding amid the city chaos.

3. Seasonally Adjusted Exercise

- Adapt Activities to the Weather: Utilize indoor options like yoga studios or gyms in colder months. In warmer months, take advantage of local parks for yoga, walking, or cycling.
- Join Community Groups: Many urban areas offer community exercise groups which can help keep you motivated while enabling you to enjoy seasonal outdoor activities.

4. Natural Element Integration

- Indoor Plants: They not only beautify your space but also help to purify the air and bring a bit of nature into your home, which is essential for balancing Vata.
- Natural Fabrics: Use natural fabrics like cotton, silk, or wool for your bedding and clothing, adapting to the requirements of each season.

5. Herbal and Natural Remedies

- Herbs and Spices: Even if you have limited cooking facilities, incorporating Ayurvedic herbs and spices into your diet can be done easily. Each season, adjust the herbs and spices you use according to Ayurvedic recommendations (like ginger and turmeric in winter or cumin and coriander in summer).
- DIY Herbal Teas: Make your own herbal teas with fresh ingredients like mint, ginger, or lemon balm which you can grow on a windowsill or balcony.

6. Seasonal Cleansing

- Detoxify Regularly: Engage in simpler forms of cleansing adapted from traditional panchakarma suited to each season. This could mean a one-day juice cleanse in spring or eating a kitchari diet for a few days in autumn.

7. Manage Environmental Stress
- Soundscapes: Use sound machines or playlists with natural sounds to create a peaceful atmosphere at home.
- Air Quality: Utilize air purifiers or introduce air-purifying plants to combat urban pollution, especially important in maintaining Kapha balance during spring.

8. Community and Social Health
- Join Ayurvedic Workshops or Groups: Look for local workshops, cooking classes, or meet-ups focused on Ayurveda which can offer support and deepen your understanding of how to live in tune with natural cycles, even in an urban environment.

By making these adjustments, city dwellers can bridge the gap between the fast-paced urban environment and Ayurveda's ancient wisdom, optimizing health throughout the seasons.

Appendix

Sr no	Name (Botanical Name)	Rasa	Guna	Vipaka	Virya	Actions
1	Agaru (Aquilaria Agallocha)	Bitter	Light, Dry	Pungent	Hot	Anti-asthmatic
2	Agnimantha (Premna Integrifolia)	Bitter, Pungent	Light, Dry	Pungent	Hot	Anti-inflammatory, diaphoretic
3	Ahiphena (Papaver Somniferum)	Bitter	Light, Dry	Pungent	Cooling	Analgesic, sedative
4	Amalaki (Emblica Officinalis)	Sour, Bitter, Astringent, Sweet	Light, Dry	Sweet	Cooling	Rejuvenative
5	Apamarga	Pung	Light,	Pungen	Hot	Diuretic,

	(Achyranth es Aspera)	ent, Bitter	Dry	t		clears obstructions ,
7	Aragvadha (Cassia Fistula)	Sweet	Heavy, Oily	Sweet	Cooling	Laxative, purgative
8	Ardraka-Sunti (Fresh & Dried ginger, Zingiber Officinale)	Pung ent	Light, Dry	Sweet	Hot	Anti-inflammator y, digestive aid
9	Arjuna (Terminali a Arjuna)	Astri ngent	Light, Dry	Sweet	Cooling	Cardioprote ctive
10	Arkadvaya (Calotropis Gigantea or Calotropis Procera)	Bitter	Light, Dry	Pungen t	Hot	Detoxifying
11	Ashwagan dha (Withania Somnifera)	Bitter , Astri ngent, Sweet	Heavy, Sticky	Sweet	Warmi ng	Adaptogeni c, anti-stress
12	Asoka (Saraca Asoca)	Bitter , Astri ngent	Light, Dry	Pungen t	Cooling	Uterine tonic, anti-dysmenorrh eal
13	Ativisha (Aconitum Heterophyl lum)	Bitter	Light, Dry	Pungen t	Hot	Anti-pyretic, digestive
14	Bakuchi	Bitter	Light	Pungen	Hot	Skin health

	(Psoralea Corylifolia)	, Pungent		t		promoter
15	Baladvayam (Sida Cordifolia)	Sweet	Heavy, Sticky	Sweet	Cooling	Strength-promoting, rejuvenative
16	Bhallataka (Semecarpus Anacardium)	Pungent, Astringent, Sweet	Light, Penetrating	Sweet	Hot	Strong anti-inflammatory, rejuvenative
17	Bharangi (Clerodendrum Serratum)	Bitter, Pungent	Light	Pungent	Hot	Bronchodilator
18	Bhrungaraj (Eclipta Alba)	Bitter, Pungent	Light, Dry	Pungent	Cooling	Hair tonic, hepatoprotective
19	Bibhitaka (Terminalia Bellirica)	Astringent	Light, Dry	Sweet	Hot	Rejuvenative, particularly beneficial for the lungs and hair
20	Bijak/ Vijaysar (Pterocarpus Marsupium)	Bitter, Astringent	Light	Pungent	Cooling	Anti-diabetic, reduces fat and cholesterol
21	Bilva (Aegle Marmelos)	Astringent, Bitter	Light, Dry	Pungent	Cooling	Digestive, anti-diarrheal
22	Brahmi	Bitter	Light,	Sweet	Cooling	Cognitive

	(Bacopa Monnieri)	, Sweet	Slimy			enhancer
23	Bruhati (Solanum Indicum)	Bitter	Light, Dry	Pungent	Hot	Bronchodilator, anti-asthmatic
24	Chandanadvaya (Red and White varieties)	Bitter , Sweet	Light, Cool	Sweet	Cooling	Skin tonic, anti-pyretic
25	Chitraka (Plumbago Zeylanica)	Pungent, Bitter	Light, Dry	Pungent	Hot	Digestive stimulant, anti-inflammatory
26	Dadima (Pomegranate, Punica Granatum)	Sweet , Sour, Astringent	Light, Dry	Sweet	Cooling	Cardiotonic, astringent
27	Devadaru (Cedrus Deodara)	Bitter , Pungent	Light, Dry	Pungent	Hot	Anti-inflammatory, anti-arthritic
28	Dhataki (Woodfordia Fruticosa)	Astringent	Light, Dry	Pungent	Hot	Fermentative, used in making medicated wines
29	Durva (Cynodon Dactylon)	Sweet , Astringent	Light, Dry	Sweet	Cooling	Hemostatic, diuretic
30	Eladvayam (Elettaria Cardamomum and	Sweet , Pungent	Light	Sweet	Cooling	Digestive, aromatic stimulant

	Amomum Subulatum)					
31	Eranda (Ricinus Communis)	Sweet , Astri ngent	Heavy, Oily	Sweet	Hot	Laxative, anti-inflammator y
32	Gambhari (Gmelina Arborea)	Bitter , Astri ngent, Sweet	Light, Dry	Sweet	Cooling	Nourishes tissue, aids in recovery
33	Gokshura (Tribulus Terrestris)	Sweet , Astri ngent	Light, Dry	Sweet	Cooling	Urinary and reproductiv e tonic
34	Guduchi (Tinospora Cordifolia)	Bitter	Light, Oily	Sweet	Hot	Immunomo dulator, anti-fever
35	Guggulu (Commiph ora Mukul)	Bitter , Pung ent, Astri ngent	Light, Dry	Pungen t	Hot	Anti-inflammator y, lipid-lowering
36	Haridradva ya (combinati on of two types of turmeric)	Bitter , Pung ent	Dry, Light	Pungen t	Hot	Anti-inflammator y
37	Haritaki (Terminali a Chebula)	Astri ngent, Sweet , Sour,	Light, Dry	Sweet	Heating	Rejuvenativ e, promotes longevity

		Bitter, Pungent				
38	Hingu (Asafoetida)	Pungent	Light, Penetrating	Pungent	Hot	Digestive stimulant, anti-flatulent
39	Jambu (Syzygium Cumini)	Astringent	Dry	Pungent	Cooling	Anti-diabetic
40	Jatamansi (Nardostachys Jatamansi)	Bitter, Astringent	Light, Dry	Pungent	Cooling	Sedative, promotes hair growth
41	Jatiphal (Nutmeg, Myristica Fragrans)	Pungent, Astringent	Light, Oily	Pungent	Hot	Sedative, aids in digestion
42	Jeerakadvaya (Cuminum Cyminum and Nigella Sativa)	Pungent	Light	Pungent	Cooling (Cumin), Heating (Black Cumin)	Digestive stimulant
43	Kalamegha (Andrographis Paniculata)	Bitter	Light, Dry	Pungent	Cooling	Hepatoprotective, immune booster
44	Kampillaka (Mallotus Philippensis)	Astringent	Light, Dry	Pungent	Hot	Purging and detoxifying
45	Kanchanar	Astri	Light,	Pungen	Cooling	Anti-

		ngent	Dry	t		inflammatory, useful in glandular swellings
46	Kantakari (Solanum Xanthocarpum)	Bitter, Pungent	Light, Penetrating	Pungent	Hot	Bronchodilator
47	Kapikacchu (Mucuna Pruriens)	Sweet	Heavy, Sticky	Sweet	Hot	Nervine tonic, increases sperm count
48	Karkatakshringi (Pistacia Integerrima)	Pungent, Astringent	Light	Pungent	Hot	Respiratory stimulant
49	Karpura (Camphor, Cinnamomum Camphora)	Bitter, Pungent	Light, Dry	Pungent	Cooling	Stimulant, decongestant
50	Katuki (Picrorhiza Kurroa)	Bitter	Light, Dry	Pungent	Cooling	Liver protective
51	Khadira (Acacia Catechu)	Astringent, Bitter	Light, Dry	Pungent	Cooling	Anti-inflammatory, skin healing
52	Kiratatikta (Swertia Chirata)	Bitter	Light, Dry	Pungent	Cooling	Anti-fever, blood purifier
53	Kumari (Aloe Vera)	Bitter	Sticky, Heavy	Sweet	Cooling	Laxative, skin healing
54	Kumkum	Bitter	Light,	Sweet	Cooling	Mood

	Kesara (Saffron, Crocus Sativus)	, Sweet	Oily			enhancer, rejuvenative
55	Kupilu (Strychnos Nux-vomica)	Bitter	Light, Dry	Pungent	Hot	Highly toxic, used in minute doses for nervous disorders
56	Kushta (Saussurea Lappa)	Bitter, Pungent	Light, Penetrating	Pungent	Hot	Anti-inflammatory, antispasmodic
57	Kutaja (Holarrhena Antidysenterica)	Bitter	Light, Dry	Pungent	Cooling	Anti-dysenteric, anti-diarrheal
58	Lavanga (Clove, Syzygium Aromaticum)	Pungent	Light, Penetrating	Pungent	Hot	Analgesic, dental pain reliever
59	Lodhra (Symplocos Racemosa)	Astringent	Light, Dry	Pungent	Cooling	Uterine tonic, beneficial in skin diseases
60	Madanaphala (Randia Dumetorum)	Pungent	Light	Pungent	Hot	Emetic, used in detoxification
61	Mandukap	Bitter	Light,	Sweet	Cooling	Cognitive

	arni (Centella Asiatica)	, Sweet	Oily			enhancer, promotes longevity
62	Manjishtha (Rubia Cordifolia)	Bitter , Astri ngent	Light, Dry	Pungen t	Cooling	Blood purifier
63	Maricha (Black Pepper, Piper Nigrum)	Pung ent	Light, Penetra ting	Pungen t	Hot	Digestive stimulant, enhances bioavailabili ty
64	Musta (Cyperus Rotundus)	Astri ngent, Bitter	Light, Dry	Pungen t	Cooling	Digestive, anti-diarrheal
65	Nagakesha ra (Mesua Ferrea)	Astri ngent, Pung ent	Light, Dry	Pungen t	Cooling	Antihemorr hagic, enhances complexion
66	Nimba (Neem, Azadiracht a Indica)	Bitter	Light, Dry	Pungen t	Cooling	Anti-bacterial, anti-viral
67	Nirgundi (Vitex Negundo)	Pung ent, Bitter , Astri ngent	Light, Dry	Pungen t	Hot	Analgesic, anti-inflammator y
68	Palasha (Butea Monosper ma)	Astri ngent	Light, Dry	Pungen t	Hot	Anthelminti c, astringent
69	Parpata (Fumaria Indica)	Bitter	Light, Dry	Pungen t	Cooling	Blood purifier, anti-pyretic

70	Pashanabh eda (Bergenia Ligulata)	Astri ngent, Bitter	Light, Rough	Pungen t	Cooling	Lithotriptic, diuretic
71	Patala (Stereosper mum Suaveolens)	Bitter	Light	Pungen t	Cool	Diuretic
72	Pippali-Pippalimul a (Piper Longum)	Pung ent	Light, Penetra ting	Sweet	Hot	Enhances bioavailabili ty of drugs
73	Prishnipar ni (Uraria Picta)	Bitter , Astri ngent	Heavy, Oily	Pungen t	Cooling	Rejuvenativ e, diuretic
74	Punarnava (Boerhavia Diffusa)	Sweet , Bitter , Astri gent	Light, Dry	Pungen t	Heating	Diuretic, rejuvenative
75	Pushkarmo ola (Inula Racemosa)	Bitter , Pung ent	Light, Dry	Pungen t	Hot	Cardiac tonic
76	Rasna (Pluchea Lanceolata)	Bitter , Pung ent	Light, Dry	Pungen t	Hot	Anti-inflammator y, analgesic, Vatahar
77	Rasona (Garlic, Allium Sativum)	Pung ent	Penetra ting	Pungen t	Hot	Antibacteria l, cardiovascu lar tonic
78	Rohitaka	Bitter	Light,	Pungen	Hot	Hepatoprote

		, Astringent	Dry	t		ctive, spleen disorders
	(Tecomella Undulata)					
79	Saireyaka (Barleria Prionitis)	Bitter	Light	Pungent	Cooling	Anti-inflammatory
80	Sarivadvaya (Hemidesmus Indicus)	Sweet , Bitter	Heavy, Sticky	Sweet	Cooling	Blood purifier, cooling agent
81	Sarpagandha (Rauwolfia Serpentina)	Bitter	Light, Dry	Pungent	Cooling	Hypotensive, sedative
82	Shalaparni (Desmodium Gangeticum)	Bitter	Light	Pungent	Cooling	Rejuvenative
83	Shallaki (Boswellia Serrata)	Bitter	Dry	Pungent	Cooling	Anti-inflammatory for joints
84	Shalmali (Bombax Ceiba)	Astringent	Light, Dry	Sweet	Cooling	Hemostatic, beneficial in menorrhagia
85	Shankhapushpi (Convolvulus Pluricaulis)	Bitter , Sweet	Light, Slimy	Sweet	Cooling	Cognitive enhancer
86	Shatavari (Asparagus	Sweet ,	Heavy, Oily	Sweet	Cooling	Rejuvenative for female

	Racemosus)	Bitter				reproductive system, Lactation
87	Shigru (Moringa Oleifera)	Bitter , Pungent	Light, Dry	Pungent	Hot	Nutritional supplement, anti-inflammatory
88	Shirisha (Albizia Lebbeck)	Bitter	Light	Pungent	Cooling	Anti-allergic, detoxifying
89	Shyonaka (Oroxylum Indicum)	Bitter , Astringent	Light	Pungent	Cooling	Anti-inflammatory, supportive in respiratory conditions
90	Talisa Patra (Abies Webbiana)	Pungent, Bitter	Light, Dry	Pungent	Hot	Respiratory stimulant
91	Tila (Sesame seeds, Sesamum Indicum)	Sweet	Oily, Heavy	Sweet	Warming	Nourishing, strengthens bones
92	Trivrut (Operculina Turpethum)	Bitter , Sweet	Light, Dry	Pungent	Cooling	Laxative, purgative
93	Tulasi (Ocimum Sanctum)	Pungent, Bitter	Light, Dry	Pungent	Hot	Adaptogenic, anti-inflammatory, promotes

						respiratory health
94	Tvak (Cinnamon, Cinnamomum Verum)	Sweet, Pungent, Bitter	Light, Dry	Sweet	Hot	Blood sugar regulator
95	Ushira (Vetiveria Zizanioides)	Sweet, Bitter	Light, Cool	Sweet	Cooling	Cooling, hydrating
96	Vacha (Acorus Calamus)	Pungent, Bitter	Light, Penetrating	Pungent	Hot	Cognitive enhancer, speech clarifier
97	Varahi (Dioscorea Bulbifera)	Sweet	Heavy, Oily	Sweet	Cooling	Anti-inflammatory
98	Varuna (Crataeva Nurvala)	Bitter, Astringent	Light, Dry	Pungent	Cooling	Lithotriptic (dissolves stones)
99	Vasa (Adhatoda Vasica)	Bitter	Light, Dry	Pungent	Cooling	Bronchodilator, anti-asthmatic
100	Vatsanabha (Aconitum Ferox)	Pungent	Light, Dry	Pungent	Hot	Potent toxin, used in very controlled doses for therapeutic purposes
101	Vidanga (Embelia Ribes)	Pungent, Astri	Light, Dry	Pungent	Hot	Anthelmintic, anti-parasitic

		ngent, Bitter				
102	Vidari (Pueraria Tuberosa)	Sweet	Heavy, Sticky	Sweet	Cooling	Rejuvenative, nourishing
103	Yastimadhu (Licorice, Glycyrrhiza Glabra)	Sweet	Heavy, Sticky	Sweet	Cooling	Demulcent, anti-ulcerative
104	Yavani (Trachyspermum Ammi)	Pungent	Light, Dry	Pungent	Hot	Digestive, respiratory stimulant
105	Patha (Cissampelos pareira)	Bitter, Astringent	Light, Dry	Pungent	Cooling	Detoxifying, skin disorders, fever

B. How to Make Your Own Ayurvedic Spice Mixes

Creating your own Ayurvedic spice mixes can be a delightful way to enhance your meals, both in flavour and health benefits. These mixes are tailored to balance the doshas (Vata, Pitta, and Kapha) and can be adapted based on seasonal changes or individual health needs. Here's how you can prepare three basic Ayurvedic spice mixes at home:

1. Vata-Balancing Spice Mix

Vata is characterized by qualities of cold, light, and dryness. A Vata-pacifying spice mix generally includes grounding and warming spices that help stimulate digestion and increase circulation.

Ingredients:
- 2 tablespoons cumin powder
- 2 tablespoons ginger powder
- 2 tablespoons turmeric powder
- 1 tablespoon asafoetida (hing) powder
- 1 tablespoon salt (rock salt preferred)
- 2 tablespoons ajwain (carom seeds)
- 1 teaspoon black pepper powder

Instructions:
1. Mix all the ingredients in a bowl thoroughly.
2. Store the mixture in an airtight container away from direct sunlight.
3. Use a small amount to season dishes like soups, stews, and vegetables.

2. Pitta-Balancing Spice Mix

Pitta embodies fire and water, and it is often characterized by heat. A Pitta-pacifying spice mix should be cooling and not too spicy.

Ingredients:

- 2 tablespoons coriander powder
- 2 tablespoons fennel seeds
- 1 tablespoon cumin powder
- 1 tablespoon cardamom powder
- 1 tablespoon mint powder
- 1 teaspoon turmeric powder
- 1 teaspoon cinnamon powder

Instructions:
1. In a dry skillet over medium heat, lightly roast the fennel seeds just until they release their aroma.
2. Grind the roasted fennel seeds and the rest of the spices using a mortar and pestle or a spice grinder until finely ground.
3. Store in an airtight container in a cool, dry place.
4. Sprinkle over dishes or use in marinades to provide a cooling effect, particularly beneficial during warmer seasons.

3. Kapha-Balancing Spice Mix
Kapha is characterized by qualities of heaviness, coldness, and oiliness. A Kapha spice mix should be warming and invigorating to stimulate the system.

Ingredients:
- 3 tablespoons black pepper
- 3 tablespoons ginger powder
- 2 tablespoons cinnamon powder
- 1 tablespoon clove powder
- 2 tablespoons turmeric powder

- 1 tablespoon mustard seeds
- 1 tablespoon fenugreek seeds

Instructions:
1. Combine all ingredients in a spice grinder or mortar and pestle, grinding them into a fine powder.
2. If using mustard and fenugreek seeds, lightly toast them in a dry skillet before grinding to enhance their flavors and ease of grinding.
3. Store the spice mix in an airtight container in a cool, dry place.
4. This mix can be used in small quantities to season dishes, especially during the cold and wet seasons.

General Tips:
- Always start with the freshest spices possible for the best flavor and health benefits.
- Adjust the quantity and variety of spices based on your taste preferences and any specific health considerations.
- Use these spices to cook vegetables, grains, or legumes, or as seasoning for snacks.

These Ayurvedic spice mixes not only elevate the taste of your meals but also enhance digestive strength and help balance bodily doshas, thus contributing to overall health and wellness.

Glossary

Ayurveda, with its rich ancient wisdom, employs unique terminologies that are pivotal for understanding its principles and practices. Here are explanations of key Ayurvedic terms that will help you comprehend this traditional system of medicine better:

1. Dosha

Doshas are the fundamental bio-energies found throughout the human body and mind. They govern all physical and mental processes and provide every living being with an individual blueprint for health and fulfilment. The three doshas are Vata (air and space), Pitta (fire and water), and Kapha (water and earth).

2. Prakriti
Prakriti refers to your inherent constitution, determined at the moment of conception, which remains constant throughout life. It's a unique combination of Vata, Pitta, and Kapha, which dictates your body's natural state of balance and tendencies towards disease.

3. Vikriti
Vikriti denotes your current health condition, representing imbalances in the doshas distinct from your baseline state (Prakriti). Understanding your Vikriti is crucial for applying Ayurvedic principles to restore balance and health.

4. Agni
Agni translates to "fire," specifically the digestive fire. It is responsible for metabolizing the food and experiences into useful energy and waste. A strong Agni is vital for good health, while a weak Agni can lead to indigestion and the accumulation of toxins.

5. Ama
Ama denotes toxins that accumulate in the body due to improper digestion. These can block bodily channels and hamper normal functioning, potentially leading to disease. Keeping Agni strong ensures minimal Ama accumulation.

6. Ojas
Ojas is the essence that provides vitality, strength, and immunity. It is the final product of digestion that correlates with one's inner strength, health, and

immunity. Enhanced Ojas manifests as clarity of perception, physical strength, and immunity.

7. Dhatus
Dhatus are the bodily tissues that support the structure and functioning of the body. There are seven Dhatus: Rasa (plasma), Rakta (blood cells), Mamsa (muscle), Meda (fat), Asthi (bones), Majja (bone marrow), and Shukra (reproductive fluid).

8. Srotas
Srotas are channels through which various materials (like nutrients, water, and wastes) are transported throughout the body. Proper functioning of Srotas ensures efficient distribution of nutrients and timely elimination of wastes.

9. Chakras
In Ayurveda, chakras are considered energy centers within the body that align with specific physical, emotional, and spiritual functions. Balancing these chakras is thought to enhance well-being and health.

10. Ritucharya
Ritucharya denotes seasonal regimes. Ayurveda suggests lifestyle and dietary modifications according to seasonal changes to balance the doshic influences that naturally fluctuate with the seasons.

11. Dinacharya
Dinacharya refers to daily routines suggested by Ayurveda to align with natural circadian rhythms. These practices include waking up early, practicing yoga, meditating, and eating meals at regular times each day.

12. Panchakarma

Panchakarma, meaning "five actions," is a set of five therapeutic treatments intended to cleanse the body of toxins (Ama). It is a cornerstone of Ayurvedic medicine designed to purify the entire system and restore balance and well-being. The five main procedures are Vamana (therapeutic vomiting), Virechana (purgation), Basti (enema), Nasya (nasal administration), and Raktamokshana (bloodletting).

13. Rasayana

Rasayana refers to rejuvenation therapy in Ayurveda. It encompasses a variety of practices, including special diets, herbal remedies, massage therapies, meditation, and other procedures aimed at revitalizing the body and extending lifespan. Rasayana treatments are intended to boost immunity and vitality, thereby promoting longevity and overall health.

14. Marma Points

Marma points are vital points on the body similar to acupuncture points in Chinese medicine. Stimulating these points through touch or massage can help release blocked energy and promote healing. Marma therapy is used to treat and prevent health issues, as well as to relieve pain and improve the flow of prana (vital life force).

15. Pranayama

Pranayama refers to the practice of controlling the breath, which is the source of our prana, or vital life force. It is used in Ayurveda to restore and maintain health and to balance the doshas. Specific pranayama techniques can have cooling, warming, or balancing effects, making them useful for addressing different doshic imbalances.

16. Abhyanga

Abhyanga is the practice of oil massage, considered a daily routine in Ayurveda to maintain health and longevity. The massage is typically performed with oil infused with herbs suited to the individual's dosha. Abhyanga is known to nourish the body, promote flexibility, de-stress the mind, and detoxify.

17. Swedana

Swedana is a therapeutic treatment involving induced sweating. It is often used after Abhyanga to open pores and flush out impurities through the skin. It can be done using steam boxes, steam tents, or warm compresses, and is a common part of the Panchakarma cleansing process.

18. Ayurvedic Clock

Ayurveda divides the day into segments based on dominant doshas. Understanding this Ayurvedic clock can help in planning daily activities in tune with natural rhythms. For instance, Vata time (2-6), both am and pm, is optimal for creativity, Pitta time (10-2) for productivity, and Kapha time (6-10) for physical activities.

19. Agni Types

Agni types refer to the state of the digestive fire. It can be strong (Tikshna), weak (Manda), variable (Vishama), and balanced (Sama). Recognizing your Agni type can guide dietary choices and eating habits necessary to maintain optimal digestion and overall health.

20. Guna

In Ayurveda, everything in nature is made up of three fundamental qualities (gunas): Sattva, Rajas, and Tamas. Sattva denotes purity and clarity, Rajas refers to activity and movement, and Tamas is associated with inertia and darkness. Balancing these qualities in the mind and body supports emotional and physical health.

www.ingramcontent.com/pod-product-compliance
Lightning Source LLC
Chambersburg PA
CBHW082109220526
45472CB00009B/2111